M000268650

Readers Love This Inspiring Book!

"Sometimes, for anomaly, life creates rainbows: one is awestruck by the colors, the dance, and the rare experience as if spirits have been set free to plumb this game we call 'Life.'

Oh, the wonder of it all!

"A little girl in a barn caught in an instance of Northern Lights—AVA FRICK!—captured in her 'rainbow' of dancing kittens extrapolating the prancing of their gaits, a gated equestrian's, or a braying ass. Soon, DOCTOR AVA, conducting a symphony of life so wonderful, so necessary!

"Oh, the wonder of it all!

"One does not read these pages without profound admiration of Ronald Joseph Kule's navigation through this amazing woman's life as he tells us her story. Read these pages, my friends, and whisper, 'Thank goodness for the GODDESS AVA!'"
—**Michael D. Roberts, American Actor.**

"Ronald Joseph Kule and Dr. Ava Frick have joined to tell the truly fascinating story of what is no less than a real-life Yoda of Veterinary Medicine. Dr. Frick is a national treasure, and Kule opens the treasure trove for all of us to see."
—**John Truman Wolfe, #1 Amazon bestselling author**

"Ava Frick is a unique individual who has in-depth training from formal education and yet remained open and in continuous search of better understandings. Animals are keen to the energy and the rhythm of this truth and they have responded favorably, naturally, to the presence of her uniqueness! The flow of that rhythm and the balance of natural harmony expressed in this biography produce a dance that is pleasing to watch and fun to experience. The Ava that I know makes full use of this free-flowing dance here, and the animals she has met love her for it!"
—Dennis Cappel, horse trainer/farrier & author; Reserved Champion, 2016 Extreme Mustang Makeover in Sedalia, MO; 2016 Colt Starting Champion at the Iowa Equine Fair

"Conversations with Animals... is a really entertaining book, inspiring, too. It's the timeless story of a girl who achieves her dream. A page-turner, it delivers many humorous episodes involving pet animals as well as much promise for the future of animal healthcare and rehabilitation. Good luck, Dr. Frick!"
—Alan Griffiths, Ph.D., Professor, Salt Lake Community College, Utah

"Dr Ava Frick's holistic methods, we find in her biography, have been amazingly successful in diagnosing and treating animals which many traditional practitioners could not help. This book brings to animal lovers and professionals keen insight into how she tunes in with the animal world and listens, helps, and heals in a way like no one else."
—Angie Porter, Inventor of the FURminator

CONVERSATIONS
with
ANIMALS

From Farm Girl To Pioneering Veterinarian,
The Dr. Ava Frick Story

RONALD JOSEPH KULE
with
AVA FRICK, DVM

Foreword by
Dr. Michael W. Fox, BVetMed, Ph.D., DSc,
MRCVS

Conversations with Animals
From Farm Girl To Pioneering Veterinarian,
The Dr. Ava Frick Story
by
Ronald Joseph Kule and Ava Frick, DVM

© 2019 by Ava Frick and Ronald Joseph Kule.
All Rights Reserved.

ISBN: 978-1-7346528-4-0

Published by KuleBooks LLC
Clearwater, Florida

Cover Design: Rebecacovers

Editor: KuleBooks LLC

Printed in the U.S.A.

Table of Contents

INTRODUCTION

Animals speak to us all the time in their own ways: the movement of an ear, the flicking of the skin, swishing or puffing up of a tail, the size of the pupils, slight turns of the head, and moving toward or away from another being or pressure. They tell us plenty with posture: where the head is in relationship to the rest of the body, the top line, how the position of the legs relate or align, the gait; and, yes, bucking, kicking, scratching, and biting are all communications, all telltale invitations to dance.

Dance is communication without words—an expression similar to close associations with animals. Our task as humans is to learn from animals, to be alert and aware of their styles of communication, not only by species but by each individual. And to respond appropriately.

Using veterinary medicine, chiropractic, physiotherapy, aquatic exercise, and microcurrent therapies with animals is our way of accepting the invitation to a dance. We are asking for permission to be in their space, to grant them beingness (the right to exist as they are) and importance; to validate their feelings and expressions of concern with kindness and help; and, in the end, thank them for the opportunity, however the dance turned out.

Working with an animal the way Ava Frick, D.V.M. does—two live beings willing to "experience" and share real moments together, body-to-body and heart-to-heart; two souls co-occupying a space with affinity and agreement—is a breathtaking experience for her and for us.

"In my book, it [life] can't get too much better than that," states Dr. Frick.

Conversations with Animals… is not only a timeless tale of Dr. Frick's lifetime but also a collection of the events and animals that intimately touched and changed her. The manner in which her story is laid out is, we think, something exciting: a "Hybrid Biography," an interlacing of her biographical life story by the biographer and anecdotal stories written in Dr. Frick's own words set apart with italics and ellipses.

We believe that Doctors of Animal Chiropractic and Veterinary Medicine will find a number of informative chapters with particular appeal for helping them expand in positive ways their professional cares, healthcare concerns, and spheres of influence.

Animal lovers who own pets or business partners will, no doubt, enjoy the animal narratives.

Our overall concept is to not only showcase the extraordinary spiritual values and virtues of having live communications with other-than-human species but also reveal how Dr. Frick's unique talents enhance and define Mankind through its relations with all living species. In our view and opinion, life's essence *is spiritual.*

And endlessly fascinating!

—Ava Frick, D.V.M. and

Ronald Joseph Kule

* * *

FOREWORD
by
Michael W. Fox

This is a uniquely engaging book – part biographical, part inspirational, and intensely instructive about our relationships with and treatment of other creatures. Looking through the heart and eyes of a small girl who decided, as I similarly did, to one day be a veterinarian, we discover in *Conversations with Animals...* the power of real living. This power eludes us when we are not aware of our interspecies relationships; too often, ignorance and denial of this truth results in misunderstandings, cruelties, and suffering for the animals.

Humans and animals share a single biosphere of wonder and beauty, tragedy, and suffering. This is the reality of human/animal co-existence on Earth, of which Ava Frick was aware at a young age. She was blessed with this awareness by living on a family farm, awakening daily to the timeless communion of creatures great and small.

In the otherness of fellow creatures lies the living history and mystery of our own origins, of our DNA; yet, inherent, adaptive, survivalist wisdom and security come when we find our way, our purpose for living.

Conversations with Animals... urges us on, away from human-centeredness (anthropocentrism) toward deeper metaphysical, spiritual, and social engagements – healing relationships – with all fellow creatures, echoing the words of native American Indian Chief Dan George of the Tsleil-Waututh Nation in British Columbia.

"One thing to remember is to talk to the animals. If you do, they will talk back to you. But if you don't talk to the animals, they won't talk back to you, then you won't understand, and when you don't understand you will fear, and when you fear you will destroy the animals, and if you destroy the animals, you will destroy yourself."

Having experienced the ups and downs of a variety of animal relationships before we enrolled, Dr. Ava and I expanded our veterinary scopes and visions by actively seeking out, learning, and applying to our animal patients – later, advocating – other healing modalities used on humans (some for centuries), including herbal phytotherapy, chiropractic, massage, acupuncture, electrotherapy, rehabilitation, and Nutritionals, among others. Being long-standing members of the American Holistic Veterinary Medical Association, we know that no one treatment fits all; that each individual animal is unique.

The handling and treating of animals who are fearful, even dangerous, especially those in pain, is challenging. But Dr. Ava shares with her readers how patience, acquaintance, respect, and understanding are elemental, even essential, virtues of good veterinary practice and animal care.

As well, throughout this book, Dr. Ava's understandings accumulated through her communication with and treatment of animals in need of veterinary care are demonstrated ably under the skilled work of her biographer, Ronald Joseph Kule.

The human species can no longer afford to, if ever it could, remain ignorant of interspecies relationships. The significances and values of animals in our lives increase exponentially the more our lifestyles and workplaces disconnect us from our biological and psychological roots. All parts of life and the natural world in which we co-exist are *vital!*

Other fellow creatures have their personal displays of affection, well-being, and existential joy---their own dances to the songs of their spirits. This book is an introduction to and celebration of this reality, an understanding of which lies at the core of the ethical caring for animals, and veterinary diagnostics and healing.

Conversations with Animals... helps reconnect us to the great healing which we so urgently need in these times of existential crises facing not only humanity but all living creatures, great and small."

— Michael W. Fox BVetMed, Ph.D., DSc, MRCVS

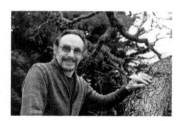

Dr. Michael W. Fox

Michael W. Fox was born and educated in the UK, earning his veterinary degree from the Royal Veterinary College London and subsequently a Ph.D. in medicine and a D.Sc. in ethology/animal behavior from the University of London. Spending most of his professional life in the USA as an advocate for animal protection, rights, One Health, and conservation, he has published over 40 books and writes the nationally syndicated newspaper columnist *Animal Doctor*. Website: www.drfoxonehealth.com

CONVERSATIONS with ANIMALS

From Farm Girl To Pioneering Veterinarian ~

The Dr. Ava Frick Story

CHAPTER 1: ROOTS

Residents of America's Midwest summer cauldron suffered 118-degree heat and high humidity on the hottest day in state-recorded history less than a year before July 4, 1955. On that date, a newborn inhaled her first gulp of life-giving air at five a.m., piercing the patchy silence of St. Francis Hospital's small nursery in rural Washington, Missouri. At the time, U.S. President Dwight David Eisenhower occupied the White House in his first term, and Frank Sinatra's *Learnin' the Blues* claimed the ears of almost everyone following *Your Hit Parade* only slightly less than Les Paul and Mary Ford's *Hummingbird*. On the nation's holiday celebrating inalienable freedoms, the infant joined an estimated 272,432 other new American babies who would live among an estimated world population of 2,782,098,943 people.

Celebrated Hollywood actress Ava Gardner advanced the popularity of her first name among most Americans by then, but the new infant's parents named their second-born daughter "Ava" simply because they liked the sound of it.

The word Ava means "origin" and "popularity." It is derived from "Avis" (Latin for "bird," or "Chava" ("life" or "living one") from the Hebrew form of "Eve." If from the Hebrew "Eve," it derives from "hawwah," which, in turn, derived from "chavvâh," means "to breathe or live; living." Ava Lee Frick's appearance served as both harbinger and accelerant to the heating up of a firestorm of notable changes that would enter the world of veterinary medicine through which she, too, would breathe life and health back into the survival potential of many types of animals. Frick's hard-won understandings and applications of the practicalities and possibilities within her primary field and those of animal chiropractic she would meld with other compassionate treatments—herbal phytotherapy, Alpha-Stim® technology, early laser-therapy design, Standard Process® whole-food supplements, hair-tissue-mineral analysis in animals, and Ayurvedic Medicine, to name a few. She would, in time, help blossom and expand their influence—hers as well—well beyond local, regional, state, and national boundaries; certainly far beyond the accepted norms of her time.

Ava's mother, Sarah Mae Cartwright, was a descendant

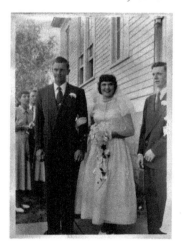

of the decidedly-British Henson clan which, decades earlier, departed from Liverpool, England and landed at New York City's Ellis Island well before Lady Liberty's torch ever lit up New York Harbor waters. She met her future husband in a dance hall in Herman, Missouri, the night his snappy military uniform and fit, six-foot-one frame caught her eye. They took to the dance floor right away. A couple of dances, a few dates, and six months later, they married. In time, Sarah birthed a daughter in the early Fifties. Eventually, three more came.

She managed her rural household and raised her girls until they attended high school, at which time she became Secretary of Union High. Years later, she occupied a womenswear position at the newly opened, local Wal-Mart store.

Ava's great-great, paternal grandfather Karl Adolphus Frick emigrated in 1857 from southwest Germany's historic Black Forest region, specifically the quaint town of Lahr. (Lahr's population census counted 6,939 residents in 1852.) Like so many others of his time, he arrived in America through Ellis Island in New York, soon ending up in Ohio for a year or so. From there, he headed west on a path most newcomers traveled in those days. In Campbellton, Missouri, he took the svelte hand of Alwine Vitt in marriage. Discovering a substantial community of German immigrants established in the rural rolling hills of eastern Missouri about 80 miles west of St. Louis, the couple settled into a residency in Franklin County far from the populous crush of St. Louis' big-city living on the banks of the unpredictable waters at the confluence of the Missouri and Mississippi rivers.

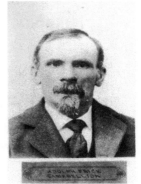

Karl Adolphus Frick, Ava's Great-great Grandfather

"Captain" Adolphus Frick later fought in our nation's oxymoronic 'Civil' War at a time Missouri was considered a divided territory claimed by both Union and Confederate forces. His survival of that conflict further established a firm foundation for the American Frick family well before Bill Haley & His Comets' *Rock Around the Clock* torched radio airwaves with a new brand of music called Rock 'n Roll in the month of Ava's birth.

The Frick family farm sat on a country hillside amid white hawthorn blossoms, flowering dogwoods, wild purple orchids, and summer orange butterfly weeds just beyond the village limits of Union, a town built by local people of faith.

The Captain's great-grandson Dennis Owen Frick, smitten by Sarah's charms and by now honorably discharged, traded military KP duty for oversight of the quarter-of-a-century-old family business operated on a spread of hundreds of acres populated with large and small farm animals. Succeeding earlier generations, Dennis became a respected denizen of the meat-packing industry in eastern Missouri. And, Ava Frick's father.

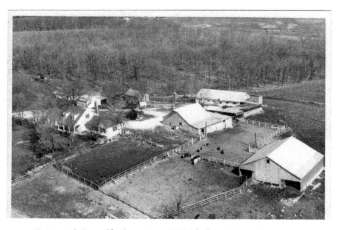

Paternal Grandfather Owen Frick's farm in Union, MO

* * *

According to astrologers, Ava's birth numbers were seven and four. Her birth year made her Life Path "lucky" number four. In one sweep, they augured growth, building, and foundation; in other words, her heritage and her pedigree fit well with what others, later, would recall as her "… practical beingness, down-to-earth outlook, and strong ideas about what is right and what is wrong."

Yet, like her birth-flower the Larkspur, this new arrival, at first, came to display unusual and accessible openness to animals, only later to people. With time, her will to give and share with animals merged with human concerns. Her distinctively pragmatic disposition, assisted and guided her through hard times and personal obstacles and helped her attain the lofty goals she envisioned almost from birth. Merely three short years past her nativity, Ava already knew her purpose in life was to work with and care for large and small animals.

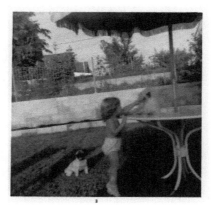

Ava at 2-3 years with Siamese cat and Pug dog

"... that purpose just WAS ...
[there's] not a lot to tell. It just was always
there, like that was why I was put on Earth
to be an animal doctor."

In 1961, a six-year-old Ava entered kindergarten at Union R10 Public School, District K—a formidable two-story, brick structure sporting plenty of windows but no air-conditioning. Excited like her peers to be in the classroom, she soon watched the bloom fall off that flower because of the uncertain antics of a classmate she knew. She started to take sick in the mornings, absolutely not wanting to return to school. When there, she refused to go outside for recess, fearing one red-headed boy, Jerry Lakebrink, a cousin to one of her best friends, Nancy. Every day, Lakebrink hid behind nearby trees and, when she walked by, jumped out and kissed her!

Oh, the strange proclivities of puppy-love at such a young age!

Ava had not been around boys much. Being kissed by one was, for her, a strange and frightening affair. At first, she said nothing to her parents about the daily occurrences. Only after some prying and a private discussion with her mother did she say why she felt sick and feared going back to school. Even with that revelation, Sarah still had to plan and meet with Jerry's mother and Ava's teacher before they convinced Ava that it was safe to return to the classroom. The boy never kissed her again, but they remained schoolmates for many years.

Coincidentally, one of Sarah's friends was Shirley Lakebrink, the aunt of the young, red-haired offender. Shirley's children mirrored the birth of Sarah's girls. Ann, Nancy, Kathy, and Andrew were in the same grades as Terry, Ava, Phyllis, and Alane (Lanie). Consequently, Ava often spent time at the Lakebrink home, in which the atmosphere literally ran cold and hot, because Herb and Shirley Lakebrink owned Lakebrink Refrigeration, the local appliance store and they ran their air conditioning continuously. Also, Shirley ran her household by a set of strict rules—if you broke one, you got hit with a wooden spoon. Just the specter of a spoon-whipping wreaked havoc and raised fear in any visiting farmgirl's heart, including Ava's. (Watching out for Shirley's wooden spoon is still remembered fondly as a running joke in the town today!)

From those early events onward, right through Grade 12 and graduation in 1973, Ava and her friends bounced along familiar dusty, gravel-covered, rural roads, riding nearly the same bright-yellow school bus to the same school every weekday.

Not unlike her peers', Ava's childhood away from the classroom made for a relatively simple lifestyle, though, at times, a curious one. Early risings for chores, weekday evenings with academic study, and copious amounts of time spent among animals, including one farm dog named "Boots," who lived a solid 14 years, occupied her waking hours. Barn cats, horses, and cows coming in seasonally for feed inside the family barn offered the young girl hours of opportunities to consider what the foundational makeup of her adult life would be—itself almost a guarantee of a steady adult hand capable of handling whatever life would bring her way.

> *"My sense of myself then was that I was a kid with some sisters. I know I really liked cats ... and that I could go days without talkin' to somebody if I wanted to.*

> *"Cats themselves are very gentle creatures. Sitting and waiting, not a twitch or a flick, poised for a quick leap as soon as the mouse or bird is calculated to be in just the right position ... then, faster than thought, they go into motion.*

> *"(I realize that's a sore subject to many and I hate it, too, when a cat kills any bird other than a sparrow.)*

> *"As a kid, my trips to the barn were planned best when I could sneak away from the sisters.*

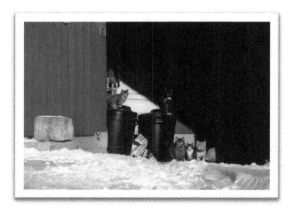

Barn cats in Winter

"Most of the barn cats were a bit wild, not a lot, but a bit. It served their purpose for survival to be that way. Some would permit me to pick them up; others not so. The best times were in the spring and summer when the new kittens ventured out from between the hay bales. Over the years, I learned that it was generally the boys who were curious and showed themselves first.

"My strategy was to be very quiet. I would be patient and sit off to the side and wait, and wait, and wait. If I could resist moving, there would soon be two, then three, and maybe four! Shortly, a game of chase and jump and spit would commence. Any unfamiliar movement, or one sly kitten realizing there was a stranger in their midst, ended my entertainment— like turning off a TV—as they skedaddled back from whence they came.

"Some days, my sister Phyllis got wind of my intent, and she would follow me, forcing me to accept that this was not going to be a great kitten-findin' day because one thing she struggled with terribly was to be quiet.

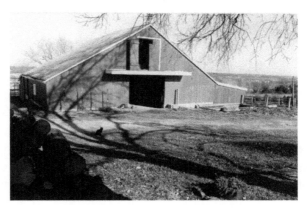

Barn with loft where Ava learned patience

"Once the kittens began to play and show themselves more, my next step was to start catchin' 'em - an opportunity to hone-in on fast, hand-eye coordination. They had to be snatched at the back of the neck, or else I would feel the impact of their claws. Because a mother cat carries her kittens this way, they will curl their back legs up and go a little limp. The innate response gave me a chance to find out if they were a boy or girl, not a simple task on kittens.

"People talk about 'puppy breath' being unique, but that can't hold a candle to the smell of a four-to-eight-week-old kitten. Aaahhh!"

* * *

Of course, Sarah rode herd over her three rambunctious young girls who, at times, forced her to gather all the energy she could muster to get her brood ready for family events away from the farm. Case in point, the time she dressed up the girls, because Dennis would come home soon to take the whole family out.

First, Sarah dressed and tidied up Ava who looked pretty in her freshly-starched and ironed white-with-light-blue-stripes outfit. She turned her attention to the other sisters while Ava wandered outside, trying to pass the time. Soon enough, a calico kitten came running by, which Ava scooped up. Cuddling it close to her face, she never expected the sudden sound and smell that erupted. The kitten had let loose a stream of diarrhea right down Ava's pristine dress! Following mixed thoughts about handling the stain herself or telling her mom, Ava turned herself in for help. The baleful look of *I can't win for losing* that overcame Sarah's face turned quickly into a command: "Take it off!" Later that evening, a satisfying *mission accomplished* flashed across Sarah's mind the second that she realized every one of her prepped girls were ready just as Dennis pulled up the driveway to the house.

To the already precocious little Ava, the lesson observed and learned from the incident was that sometimes you must do what you have to because you can; you don't wait for 'That's impossible'—something she never would forget.

In Ava's future line of work, the lesson also would come in handy in her handling of both animals and people. For the time being, however, she contently toed the line set by her parents and continued to keep mostly to herself.

* * *

Ava had three sisters: the two-years-older Terry, two-years-younger Phyllis, and the late arrival Lanie, whose antics Ava gravitated quickly toward out of amazement and amusement.

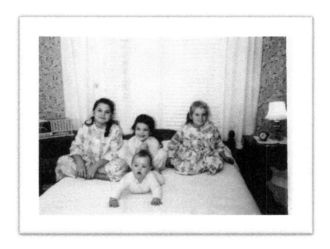

Four girls: Terry, Phyllis, Ava & Alane the baby

According to Lanie, "We played in the backyard on the old farmstead, often eating at the dinner table together in the screened-in summer house, a two-story limestone. That was before air-conditioning."

Inside the family's barn, Lanie learned how perceptive her older sister could be about animals while watching her spot with ease the young roosters from the hens among more than a dozen chickens. Later on, still amazed, she watched Ava spend hour upon hour in her room, her school books cracked open.

"Ava, why do you spend so much time studying?"

"Because I've got to be good at this so I can become an 'animal doctor,' Lanie."

Lanie figured that was the right approach and she followed her Big Sister's example, studying animals and horses from her own perspective of wanting to draw and paint them. Having found in herself an artist with a passion for communicating what went on inside her subjects, her paintings gradually reflected her spirituality more and more.

For Lanie, the disparity of their ages afforded an opportunity to watch for years how Ava's life progressed ahead of her own. In 1975, she observed how her big sister cared for her prized possessions: one, a 1962 push-button Dodge sedan that had come to her through Grandpa Frick a year earlier, and its successor, a teal-blue, 1967 Pontiac Firebird that Ava regularly cleaned and serviced.

The two vehicles were welcome alternatives that got her to and from her part-time position at the Marshall Animal Clinic. Having transportation like that meant her no longer having to bicycle three miles to and three miles back from work every day, at times under inclement Missouri skies.

Incidentally, the first veterinary student Ava ever knew, Chris Snodgrass, already was doing in that clinic the kind of work that she wanted and intended to do. Besides such affinities afforded her in that place, working there brought Ava an income, which she managed well—another work-ethic observed and admired by her younger sibling.

In fact, the smallest events in every one of the siblings' lives eventually shaped and revealed each sister's character more and more, including Ava's ever-increasing tenacity to persist through good times and bad.

But, we get ahead of her story. Let's scale back to earlier times.

* * *

CHAPTER 2: EARLY FARM LIFE

"Growing up on a farm had its ups and downs. I never knew the stress of having to plead for a pet. There were always plenty of animals to play with or observe. We were, however, short on neighbors - no extra kids with which to play - so, either I got along with my two other sisters, Terry and Phyllis, or I went to the barn and hung out with the animals.

"As it went, I was in the barn a lot! That's when I began learning to see life from the animals' eyes. I saw how they looked when scared, angry, and fierce, or they were just pretending to be. It was in their eyes, postures they took, the directions that they moved ... where the head was positioned, how the ears flicked ... the size and motion of the tail. And the sounds they made with emotions, each unique to different species. Snorting, blowing, howling, barking, braying, bellowing, clucking quietly, crowing loudly, and, yes, purring - that contented sound of a cat's purr, especially from a mother with kittens.

*"This is where the animal stories
really begin for me. For much of what I
was, growing up, came from the lessons I
learned from animals. They taught me
love, laughter, compassion, patience,
communication, value, and responsibility;
survival, caution, how to think, to share, to
admire, and to empower; companionship,
forgiveness, and that not everyone likes
you; how to be a warrior and ... death—
the most difficult. It started when I was
seven."*

* * *

Ava's grandfather and his immediate family were enterprising people. She admired the gregariousness of her Grandma Mildred Beyersdorf Frick, who regularly hosted Bridge, Garden, and Federated Club meetings in her home, accompanied by tea and hors d'oeuvres, finger sandwiches, homemade pastries, and smatterings of the German language. Occasional eavesdroppers like Ava and her sisters learned by listening.

And then there was Aunt Emma, who loved to play Canasta marathons, and who taught Ava how to play card games.

Concurrently, Grandpa Owen held his own at regular poker-night get-togethers in the cellar, replete with Cracker Barrel cheese, hard salami, crackers, and seasonal imbibements—lucky guests would earn an occasional glass, or two filled to the brim with homemade wine usually reserved for the most prominent businessmen of Union.

The makeup of the four-seasons ventilation system in the old farmhouse conveniently placed heating vents in the floors. These permitted not only cigar smoke and laughter to drift up to the scrunched-up noses and willing ears of the young children in the house but also, once the evenings got rowdy, some ear-burning language which on more than one occasion forced the girls to early bedtimes whenever Sarah also overheard those particular words!

> *"We lived next door to Grandma and Grandpa. Literally, only a door separated our home from theirs. That was until I was in the fourth grade when we moved to Prairie Dell Road. With three active Germans around us all the time, there was a heavy influence, and I grew up seeing that one <u>worked</u>. Somewhat strapped to that German workhorse outlook, I saw that [the virtues of] responsibility and productivity paid off."*

Ava's father Dennis managed Hereford and Angus cattle and operated a slaughterhouse business right on the farm—a family tradition ever since 1896 when Grandfather Edward Frick established Frick's Quality Meats. With it, he satisfied his urge to care for his family's needs as well as those of the surrounding community. By playing his role in the local culture, he shared with farmers and townspeople the venerable tradition of helping each other survive come what may.

Like most cattlemen, Dennis' heart beat with love for life and had a healthy respect for his animals. He saw to it that they were fed and raised correctly. Yet, when the time came to bring his livestock to their higher purpose in the circle of life, he switched off his emotions and orchestrated the necessary slaughtering that provided food at home and in-town at the local Frick's Market grocery.

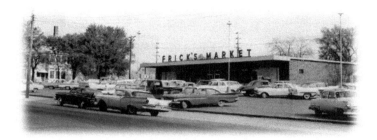

New Frick's Market, 1955

Ava was a second-grader in school and seven years old the day Grampa Frick gifted her with her first pup, which came from a litter of Welsh Corgis offered to him at his store. Upon seeing the puppy, Sarah promptly exclaimed, "Oh my, look at that little fanny she's got! Let's call her 'Fanny.'" When the daughters jumped up, excited and happy about the name, it stuck.

Fanny liked to share bubble baths whenever her young human companions sat in the farmhouse's large, warm-water-filled, claw-footed tub and took turns gingerly tossing soap bubbles into the air. In turn, the entertained sisters took delight every time the diminutive canine jumped up and down, attempting to pop them.

For Ava in particular, innocent fun filled her days throughout regular school hours and evening home chores— classroom times whiled away drawing imaginary cats with her friend Debra Mills after they completed their school assignments. The teacher, Mrs. Curtwright, set up long rectangular tables in her classroom, at which six students could sit across from each other—three on each side. Debra and Ava strategically chose to sit next to each other often, specifically to enable their creating artworks together.

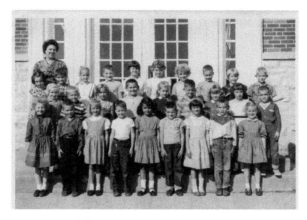

Mrs. Curtwright's second-grade class, 1962. Front row: Debra Mills first on left; Pat Johannaber last on right; Ava middle of middle row

One day a couple of months after receiving her new puppy, Ava, returning home in a happy mood after spending creative time with Debra asked, "Mom, where's Fanny?"

Sarah replied reluctantly that Fanny had been "run over."

"Is she dead?" Ava asked, tears trickling down her cheeks.

"Yes, she died."

"Well, where is she?"

"Dad took care of her."

"Well, can I see her?"

"I don't know that you'll be able to."

Dennis wasn't talking openly about Fanny' demise, leaving Ava to surmise the worst, as any youngster might do.

Each of the Frick girls had witnessed the slaughtering process previously since Dennis never hid it from them. He had their future well-being in mind when he let them watch, wanting them to know farm life and rural living as it is and to grow into women who could care for themselves no matter what happened. He knew that seeing and accepting the "bad" of life with the "good" would make them stronger in the long run. Since this was Ava's first incident of such a personal loss, however, the lingering, nagging pain lasted *years* because of the unanswered mystery attached to her hurt feelings. What hurt more than anything else was that she never had a chance to say good-bye to Fanny before the disposal of the body.

In the past, Ava never wanted to venture alone or with her sisters beyond the barn and behind the slaughterhouse building where, they were sure, they would witness the offal of animals thrown there to decompose. And she didn't go there now. Mercifully, regrettably, she never saw the remains of her prized Fanny.

Perhaps in part as recompense, a couple of years later, Sarah's brother, Uncle Dale Cartwright, an American Legion baseball player and Ava's initial impetus for a lifelong interest in St. Louis Cardinals baseball, and his wife ("Aunt Pat") gave Ava a 10-week-old, Collie-mix puppy for

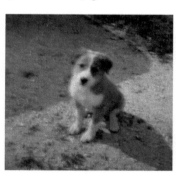

Blossom

her birthday. Ava promptly named the pup "Blossom" because of her large oval brown eyes, perky collie ears, white breast, and burnt-sienna fur.

However, this new relationship would be cut short, too. About four months later, Dennis took Blossom to a veterinarian to be spayed, and the young dog overdosed on the anesthetic Pentobarbital, ending up dead on the surgery table. Again, Ava's heavy heart skipped a beat, having been dealt another crushing blow. Ava missed saying good-bye again.

The veterinarian in nearby Beaufort, Doc Hervey, to whom Blossom had been taken, felt terrible about the outcome. After all, she had died in his clinic. Hervey brought Ava a five-month-old, small-breed, terrier-mix puppy named "Patch" because of a single dark spot over one eye. Unfortunately, Patch's habit of howling at the moon late at night disturbed Dennis (and Grampa). They acted in concert with dispatch.

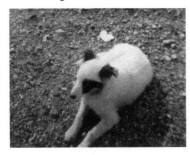

Patch

Ava was starting to identify a pattern across the string of incidents involving her pet losses. This last one made her take action. She confronted her father. Dennis didn't deny his hand in Patch's disappearance. Rather than fix the dog's problematic behavior, he had opted to get rid of him. Again, what irked Ava most was the denial of her right to see and talk with the animal one last time.

"That one made me more of a cat person. I was having so much trouble with my dogs. Also, I retreated from my dad and was less in communication with him for years after."

* * *

The following year saw mixed events for Ava. Dennis bought her a pony of her own. Up to then, she never had any riding lessons. What she knew about how to ride was limited to what she saw of Grampa and Dennis riding on the farm, and by viewing then-popular western shows on television: *Gunsmoke*, *Bonanza!,* and the *Roy Rogers Show.*

1965 was also the year Ava almost died in April. She rode her new pony in circles in the yard near the house for some time that day, pushing Dennis to shout, "Why are you only riding in the yard, Ava? Take him into the fields."

"I like riding him here."

She felt safe and comfortable in the saddle in the yard only.

"Take him out to the field, Ava."

Reluctant to venture past the yard's gate, she knew Dennis wasn't going to stop pushing.

> *"I was happy and content to ride my pony around the yard. Remember, I had never had lessons before,"* she recalled.

Ava capitulated to her father's wish. Seeing that her mom was also looking on, she steered the pony to the gate and beyond it out into the field. Feeling decidedly nervous, she had not gone far when, suddenly, a covey of birds sprang up into the air ahead of her pony. Spooked by whatever, her equine mount abruptly turned and bolted toward the barn, thinking only about its safety and, for sure, not wanting a rider onboard! Here was his chance to fall back to the familiarity of the barn he knew. His sudden about-face and gallop forced his now-terrified rider to hang on for her dear life, screaming the whole 200 yards back to the gate. Before pony and rider reached his intended goal, however, he turned on a dime and stopped just as fast—maybe because he saw Ava's parents rushing toward him?

Although the pony's motion forward stopped, Ava's momentum threw her whole body forward over his mane and head. She hit hard against the chicken-wire fence ahead of them, landing in an awkward position on top of a one-by-four board at the bottom.

Hurt and knocked (apparently) unconscious, Ava immediately went "out"—not passed but spiritually exterior from her body. She found herself observing her stilled and critically wounded body from about 30 feet above and off to one side. She watched her distressed parents lean over the apparently lifeless body of their daughter, the pony standing right beside them.

Ava had no way to communicate and let them know that she was alright because she was disconnected temporarily from the motor controls of the body. The profound experience, she knew, was altering the course of her life forever; a door had opened to another reality she sensed as something long forgotten—one in which, she realized, she was capable of making new decisions (called by some, "postulates") about what her life could be like if she survived this physical mishap.

> *"I was forever changed. From that incident forward, a part of me never forgot. I was eager to reclaim the state after I'd moved back into my body and awakened if that were possible. Also, I somehow understood anew that animals had minds of their own in a genuine sense, which served to make me more certain than ever about my purpose to not only help animals but also to understand them better."*

In the weeks that followed, Ava's body ended up with a black eye, the skin of her back peeled off (denuded), a greenstick (partial) fracture of her right radius (forearm), and a severe concussion that required two weeks of mending before she returned to school. At least, at home, she could listen to music—often her Mom's big-band music and musicals, or Disney-production songs, and other pop-music wonders. On television, the "King of the Cowboys," Roy Rogers, was a favorite of hers.

Wearing for six weeks a Medi-splint on her arm, upon her return to school, she was ridiculed for her slow-to-fade, blue-black, greenish shiner.

The pony was never seen or heard from again.

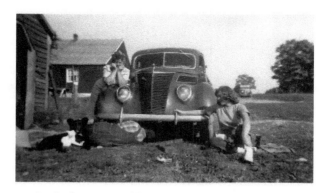

On the farm in Gerald, circa 1949. Eli (Grampie) under car; Della (Gramme) on a fender; Sarah (Mom) to the right with kittens in her lap

In better times, Ava fared well at her maternal grandfather's side in nearby Gerald. After the Cartwright family farm sold early in 1967, Grampe Eli and Gramme Della moved into a new place inside Union town limits. There. she spent more of her free time in his milieu. The man's passion for cars, motors, and engines rubbed off on the impressionable 12-year-old, developing in Ava a new and lasting affinity for all things automotive, quite in addition to her animal affairs.

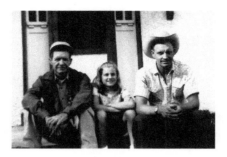

Eli, Ava, Dennis (Dad)

Ava's collaborations with her Grampe Cartwright remained in full swing up to December 1967. Just as the Frick and Cartwright families executed last-minute plans for a large gathering at his place for the coming Christmas holiday, Grampe unexpectedly died on the 24th—he had been taking nitroglycerin tablets for a heart condition never explained to the younger set. Once again, Ava faced more death bereft of any chance to say good-bye, this one far more personal for her. Yet, she was not alone in her distraught condition this time. Each family member reacted differently to the event, including her sister, Terry, whose reaction only exacerbated the grief-stricken Ava's sense of loss by telling her, "You're just carrying on"… almost adding a callous, "Get over it!"

Not too many weeks later, Ava's world scored another note of hurt in her seventh-grade school year. She broke her left arm while attending a roller-skating birthday party for Pat Johannaber, a friend.

"Guys were sticking their legs out as people skated by, and I, not knowing they were doing it, was one of their targets. I hit the hardwood floor hard, despite trying to catch myself on the way down. I knew instantly it was broken. The party was halted, and I went home. I went to the

*doctor the next day. He x-rayed my left
arm and put a cast on it."*

Of course, people do react differently to their personal mishaps, depending on their ability or inability to confront evil or death. For sure, life and death bring out strong emotional responses from us all, but we must "live and learn" by them. At any given moment, we all do what we think is the right thing to do, often learning if it was right or wrong only by the opinions of others that cause us to take another rear-view look. But, for Ava, this event piled more emotions on top of earlier losses. Still acutely aware of the harsh impact of not being allowed to say good-bye to those she loved dearly, she absorbed her personal loss and tried to move on; however, the residue of her earliest harsh experiences pressed indelibly upon her psyche, not all to the bad. She found herself better prepared not only for self-preservation but also to face and help children confront the horrendous possibility, or reality, of their animals and pets turning sick and dying, or having to be put down. She vowed to make at least a part of her life's mission the enabling of parents to be more aware of this kind of loss effect upon their children. Facing possible euthanasia for a sick or dying pet, she discussed with them <u>from her perspective and experience</u> how they could help their child work through terrible losses, which she knew only too well they would experience.

*"There was a "place" where I would
go when it was time to talk to a family
about helping their kids to say good-bye.
Not a place in this universe ... an area
within myself, an inner cosmos maybe.
Without sharing my experiences directly, I
merely told them that I knew in the future,
it would be necessary for their children to
have the opportunity to say good-bye, in
whatever way they may want. And that this*

moment should not be made light of or overlooked. It might be the night before, explaining what was about to happen and, while sitting with their pet, talk about what fun they had or a special event in the past that they shared. And if one chose to be quiet, that was OK, too. They may want to draw a picture, or make a time capsule and put a remembrance from every one of the family into it, and then at the right time have a little ceremony and bury the time capsule in the yard with the ashes or near a place where the pet liked to sit and sunbathe. But, above all, they would need the ability to say the last good-bye.

"Parents, you have to be strong and hold back your emotions as much as possible for two reasons: One, to not impose on your kids a level of sadness they may not feel or see in the passing, for, in doing so, that might shed doubt on their level of caring or love. Two, if you choose to stay with the pet as it is being euthanized, especially for dogs, this loyal companion has stood by you and had the responsibility of taking care of you. I have seen how difficult it is for the pet to leave spiritually when the owner is grief-stricken and morose. You must be strong, try really hard not to cry; instead, assure them they did a wonderful job, that it is safe to go, and that you will be OK. Don't let the flood of tears start until they are gone."

* * *

Worsening or aggravating the volatile situation, Terry, the oldest sibling, took to hollering and banging things around in response to the dramas going on around her. Like a smoldering ember, on any given day she was capable of mood swings and prone to burst out in flames if prodded too much. If a stiff breeze fanned her sister the wrong way, Ava herself could get caught in the middle of the hurricane!

For Ava, these chains of events made her childhood years radically different than those of her more mature years. Her lifestyle, by choice, revolved mostly around the animals she knew and with whom she spent time. Her reality and affinity were, in her words, *"... greater with the animals than with humans."* If others in her family did not understand her, she simply went to the barn and spent time there with the cats and dogs, and other, larger animals. However, whenever possible and while pretending to be the "animal doctor" handling animals inside the screened-in porch "veterinary clinic," time spent with her sisters was a day when everything came together for her.

* * *

To his credit, under Dennis Frick's taciturn manner and *apparently* heartless actions beat a heart of gold. He was, after all, the loyal husband, father, and hard-worker ... also, the possessor of a proud German-warrior personality well-suited to the rigors of an infamous German folk legend from long ago, in which a German knight/warrior is said to have taunted 1,000 of his enemies to cross a river separating them to fight him. After he had successfully goaded his opposition, he defeated every last one single-handedly!

Winning—more, not losing—is a known trait shared proudly among all Germans, notwithstanding the last world war's outcome. And winning with a heart full of a rich and weathered love disguised under a stolid exterior and overworked, hardened hands was Dennis' primary way to show his loyalty, fealty, and respect for his family!

The counterpoint to her husband, Sarah, brought fresh perspectives to the rural Frick family lifestyle. For one, she loved babies. She married at age 18 and birthed her daughters at 19, 21(Ava), 23, and 28. A warm-hearted mother, Sarah always made time for her girls and cared for them openly. She was the one guiding them to be better women, making sure they had extra-curricular experiences after school—tap dancing, birthday parties, and getting them to swim lessons every summer—whatever they wanted to do,

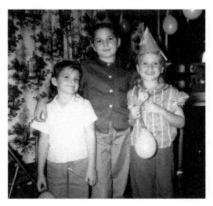

Phyllis, Terry & Ava at Terry's 9th birthday party, 1962

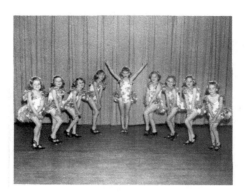

Tap dancing recital, Ava first on left

Dennis was around, but his children really didn't have a lot of one-on-one time with him.

> *"Mom was the one smoothing things over and 'Keeping the Peace.' If a person could be put next to a definition of a word in the dictionary, Mom would be placed next to KIND. She always can see things from someone else's perspective and never has been a critical person. She would consider why another might be acting or talking in a less than optimal way. She was and is the KINDEST, most CONSIDERATE person I have ever known."*

Sarah's skills inside the household complemented and matched the carpentry, welding, butchering, and groundskeeping duties of her husband. As parents, they were both skilled at whatever tasks they took on to do.

Dennis, at odd times, did find occasions to play a game of catch or croquet with his family, now and then, if not enough times to suit Ava's wishes during her growing years.

"In high school, we got a ping pong table, and Dad was fun. That was after he was not under Grampa's roof and was more independent. Lanie was five years old then, and he could see how quickly we were growing up."

No secret that all was not a bed of roses between Ava and her father. While he might mean well, he could come off as somewhat of an oppressor to her plans, although not the only one.

"Ava, you'll never be able to be a veterinarian because you'll never be able to do what has to be done" was a view echoed by her Grandma Frick on one occasion—an apparent reference to Dennis' having to end lives, not just nurture them. Ava's solution to this was to not tell either of them about her plans—a decision she would, later in her life, realize had not been the most pro-survival choice. But, at her young age, what seemed to be the right thing to do was to curtail communication.

Sister Terry, being the eldest of all the daughters, had different expectations thrust upon her. At that time, rural life and the American culture expressed a different set of values than today's. Back then, siblings toed the line set by their parents. Yet, among sibling interactions, imagination was the most valuable commodity when it came to play and friendship.

Within the Frick family, Phyllis was the primary musician, often using pliers—her "talkers"—and other available tools to bang on pots and pans and drums. (Eventually, Sarah gifted her with wooden spoons to beat on softer containers, sparing deafness to the others' ears.) Phyllis harbored a dream to play the piano like Liberace ever since her third school grade. When after several months she had not accomplished that end, she wanted to quit, but Sarah kept her going. And she did become a remarkable pianist.

Even though Ava took lessons, she never got to the point where she could sit down and play without music in front of her the way Phyllis could. Phyllis, having memorized many pieces, including Chopin and Rachmaninoff, among others, could entertain anytime and anywhere, being facile with the keyboard. Her talent came to her naturally, always making her a good guest-turned-artist at get-togethers when the conversations slowed. Phyllis was also the one who often made up funny stories with which she regaled her sisters loudly, forcing Dennis and Grandpa to joke that they wished she would take up the violin, "… because then she would have to shut up for a while."

Her other loves? More percussion instruments, the harp, stage plays, Shakespeare, and knitting.

"She can even knit socks!"

(Easier for her than darning holey ones, apparently.)

Ava played some piano, but the flute remained her forte until, years later, she drifted to harmonica on horse trails and campfire settings.

Lanie simply loved drawing horses from "eye," as well as sea life. Ever unable to find a horse to draw at rodeos, she made do with the bulls as her subjects.

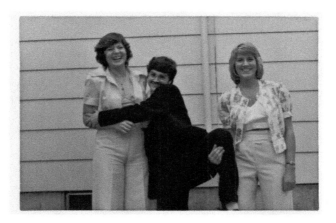

Phyllis the Thespian as Groucho Marx

While Phyllis, the acknowledged thespian of the clan, invented dramas designed to entertain her sisters, if not raise a laugh or two, Lanie was the one who, though the youngest, connected most with Ava spiritually and had a calming effect upon her whenever she needed one.

In exchange, Ava offered her siblings a keen business sense right from her younger years. She credits Grandpa Frick's influence, because he ran the grocery store, handled the money, taught Ava how to count back the change correctly when selling grapes, and sat on the United Bank of Union founding board of directors. Ava's "hobby," as she put it, offered her another outlet, as well as unexpected returns at different junctures of good and bad times.

"Even young, I was thinking of ways to make money. In the third and fourth grade, Mom would take me to town so I could go up and down the streets, selling boxes of greeting cards. People would look through a booklet, pick out what they wanted, and give me cash or a check. I

would put in the order and then deliver the
cards back to them at a profit."

By the seventh grade (1967-68), having observed Ava's privately burgeoning, enterprising ways and her continued interest in animal care, Gramme gifted her with a set of dog clippers so she could learn how to properly groom dogs. Thus, Ava practiced cutting hair on her grandmother's dog Peppy, saving the elderly relative some money at the groomer. When Ava eventually solicited for outside dog clients, her inclinations and hobby became a tidy business model that expanded and served her well for more than four decades.

"It was tough to be really good at it. It
took a lot of patience and was difficult to
manage without a real professional set
up."

The resourceful teenager continued earning enough income to stash aside some Reserves, enabling her to play "banker" with her sisters.

"I had a little nest egg goin'. My
sisters would come to me for money. I
would ask what it was for and how and
when they would be payin' me back. You
see, they had no jobs..."

Her formal backlashes hurt their relations only a little— the sisters would call Ava "stingy" for expecting to be repaid, but that never deterred them from returning to "the bank," as they named her service, anytime they had a need.

Ava's bottom line? She never shirked an opportunity to work.

"I did some babysitting. Then, at 15,
when Dr. Curtman came to town, I was

*one of his first employees at the Union
Veterinary Clinic. I have worked at Six
Flags Over Mid-America, Purina Farms,
and at an Italian restaurant, Two Guys
From Italy, as a 'waitress'—what we were
called back then."*

On one occasion, Dr. Curtman invited Ava to ride with him on a trip to Columbia, Missouri. She was excited about

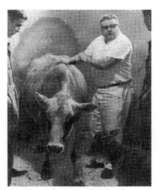

Dr. Joseph T. McGinity & cow

the opportunity to actually go to the site of her dreams, the Veterinary College. That day, she chanced to meet in his office a rather large and jolly Irishman with prominent jowls. Almost always wearing a white clinic shirt and pants, Dr. Joseph T. McGinity was a large animal clinical professor at the University of Missouri's College of Veterinary Medicine—a real treat for the farmgirl wanting to become an "animal doctor."

As Dr. Curtman and Ava departed McGinity's office, she turned and looked straight at the kindly Irishman and said, *"Keep a spot for me; I'll be back one day."* Ava walked away wearing an ear-to-ear smile for the rest of the day: McGinity had smiled proudly back, thinking without any doubt *this one, indeed, will keep her word.*

* * *

CHAPTER 3: CIRCLES OF FRIENDS

Outside of the Frick household, there were friendships to be forged. The children in the area attended the same schoolhouse classes for 12 years, and familiarity began early among different sets of students. Academic prowess and intelligence-quotient (I.Q.) scores set apart Ava's group, but they never formally "named" themselves the way other cliques did—the beauty-queen "Mannequins" and the rural/farm bunch known as "Aggies." The closest branded name applicable to Ava's group would sound a lot like the National Honor Society. In fact, there was am NHS branch in the local high school in which those named here would eventually play their parts, their GPAs being their badges of honor: Nancy, Alice, Barb, Debra, and, of course, Ava.

Debra Mills and Ava—the same duo who drew imaginary cats together—first met in kindergarten at the Union public school, a grouping of not more than 30 kids. Her mother often chaperoned sleepovers that were commonplace at her house, often with the music of the Beach Boys, the Beatles, Lulu, and Herman's Hermits playing whenever Ava controlled the record player or radio. Most indoor evening activities, including trying on makeup and dancing to the music recorded on vinyl records, took place in the large basement under the house. On most sunny summer days, the Mills' backyard swimming-pool patio was the place to be seen since no classes meant not having to worry about homework or scoring high marks on reports graded by the local teachers. Coincident to birthdays, like Ava's, fun nighttime activities centered around lighting fireworks, including cherry bombs, Roman candles, and assorted other firecrackers—*"the good stuff"*—lit mostly on the street outside the Mills' house.

The collective thread holding gathered parents of the community together while their daughters played was all of the adults involved in one way or another running local businesses. (The White Rose Café today continues to be a thriving business where generations of locals gather for down-home meals and friendly gossip and conversation.)

Ava's fourth-grade physical mishap was offset, in part, by her beginning a friendship with a new girl whose family moved from Springfield to Union. Melanie Luker found it difficult to assimilate into the mélange of student cliques at the school, but Ava right away approached her in a "friendly, sweet" way, not like the girl groups at school and in the neighborhood who were mean to the "new girl."

Melanie's family moved around a lot up to that point. "We made 12 moves by the time I was 13 years old."

Her parents were house flippers, remodeling newly acquired houses and renovating them as fast as they could. Consequently, they moved a lot. In fact, Melanie and Ava had only broken-in their friendship when the Luker family moved again. This time, though, both girls stayed in touch and remained so well into their high-school years, despite attending different schools once Melanie lived in the countryside near Gerald and attended a school in nearby Owensville.

"I remember that Ava and I shared a book, *The Velveteen Rabbit*, which we checked out from the fourth-grade bookshelf. [Written by the British author Marjory Williams, the novel tells a tale about a stuffed rabbit's imaginary wish to be real, inspired by the love of his owner.] It became a special book for us."

Melanie also recalled times she visited Ava at her farm: "… Animals … cows, horses, dogs, cats, and kittens seemed to be everywhere, and they followed Ava around like she was the Pied Piper. Like most friends do, we laughed, and we cried, and we crafted together. Ava liked crafting, not that we always had all of the supplies we needed. But, I recall Ava making glue for her projects out of mixed flour and water."

Could those hours of craft projects shared between Melanie and Ava have sparked Ava's imagination and inspired her, years later, to perfect surgical procedures that minimize time and blood loss during neutering surgeries on dogs and cats? In part, yes, but mostly because Ava spent considerable time learning to operate a sewing machine.

> *"I started sewing as a very young girl*
> *with my Grandma. Grandma was a*
> *painter, very artsy-crafty, and also a*
> *gardener. I got my first sewing machine in*
> *the 4th grade for Christmas … and did*
> *embroidery and crewel then."*

"Ava was, to me, an advanced thinker back then, and today she seems to be in a league of her own, changing aspects of her industry," opined Melanie.

Still, the two girls' parents loved their daughters, leading them to make the necessary trips to and fro between Union (where Ava lived) and Gerald about 18-20 miles away, at times with Hercules, a sharp, smart terrier mixed breed, and Sampson, part collie who bumbled around seemingly a bit dumb.

Alice Jenny and Ava connected through their Presbyterian Sunday School classes and related activities.

Alice sang in the choir, but Ava did not. When not visiting there, Ava spent time with her friend at the Union Saddle Club, of which Grandpa Frick was a founding member and which sponsored horse shows and 4H Club events.

High-school days turned into sleepover nights occasionally held at the Frick's farmhouse; others took place in Alice's house inside of Union's town limits. While the distance was not too far, about six or seven miles only, reliance on a willing parent or two depended on the weather or the season to plan and make these events. The idea of exchanging expected courtesies for the sake of the girls' safety underlay the adults' tacit agreement. Living rural and surviving the elements, after all, depended upon cooperation among all neighbors facing the same daily difficulties or seasonal complications—the trade-off for the freedoms afforded by the lifestyle.

Among fun things to do back at the farm, jumping again and again from the hayloft into fresh mounds of hay stored in the barn was a favorite pastime. Ava and her girlfriends enjoyed grand times there more than occasionally, including those with allergies to hay dust. When not hayloft jumping, Alice's fallback was riding horses. Her horse Pattycake, a cross between a Shetland pony and a draft horse, came with a white-dappled coat. Laughed and sneered at by owners of more expensive and statuesque equines because she was not much to look at, Pattycake literally out-performed many of her competitors much to the chagrin of those "equine cognoscenti" grazing the crowded venues like cattle searching for greener pastures. Alice's two other prized-possessions, Valley Star and Rimbo Badge, were quarter horses that often made hay on the horseshow circuit when ridden by Alice.

* * *

Thanksgiving 1966 presented to the Frick family a new set of twin Hereford calves. Unfortunately for the second calf, the cow would not accept it, as sometimes happens. Fortunately for Ava and Terry, however, their Dad offered the calf to them *if* they would take care of him, which meant getting up every morning to bucket-feed him before the school bus arrived at 6:45. Undaunted by the clock, the sisters excitedly took on the opportunity, naming their calf "Pilgrim," of course, because he came to them on Thanksgiving!

On alternating days, one or the other sister stepped down into the twilight-lit basement, scooped powdered milk replacer from its container, and poured it into an empty bucket, which then was filled to a specific line with warmed water. An egg whipper and some elbow grease applied vigorously took care of any clumps. In winter, bundling-up time added to the chore. Missouri winters can rise to 50-60 degrees for a few days once in a while, but mostly the temperature hovers between 40 and subzero (with wind chill factored in).

The trek to the barn ran the length of a football field. With the heavy bucket steaming through not-quite-sunlit mornings (on good-weather days), the girls took turns trudging to the barn, trying not to spill any of the precious milk as the bucket periodically banged into their legs. Entering the barn, the smell of hay and cattle greeted their nostrils, as a few cats scampered hither and yon in search of tasty morning morsels. The girls' reward for all this effort was to watch as Pilgrim's round eyes brightened and his tail switched.

Once Pilgrim got the hang of the idea that this was his new mother's udder, the challenge was to get the bucket hung on the stall panel before he anxiously took hold of the nipple. Next, the sister present sat back and listened to the specific sound the nursing bucket made with each suck as the milk ebbed and flowed into the calf's mouth until gravity gave forth nothing more of that meal. After a few weeks, Pilgrim had grown strong enough to treat the bucket like a punching bag, butting it between gulps the same way all calves do to their poor mothers.

Pilgrim did well with his motherless, young life. Terry and Ava were fond of him, but Ava especially felt attached. When the time arrived to send him out with the herd, she negotiated for more barn time. Agreed upon, the new arrangement included Ava's joining 4-H Steermanship to learn how to halter, lead, groom, and show Pilgrim in local fairs the following summer, which created opportunities for her and Dennis to do things together. As well, Bass Sibole, a friend of the family skilled in showing cattle, became her mentor and guide.

Ava made new friends through 4-H. Monthly meetings held in the old brick, one-room schoolhouse up the road from their farm made for new activity, mutual excitement, and unity among her peers there.

The year passed too soon, but the strapping 18-month-old Pilgrim and 12-year-old Ava were more than ready to

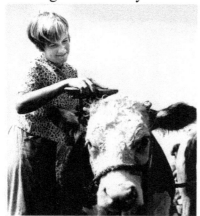

Ava & Pilgrim at Franklin County Youth Fair, 1967

take up the challenge and vie to win the Beef/Steer Showmanship Award at the Franklin County Youth Fair.

While most contestants slept on cots next to their livestock under the big tents, Ava's parents did not permit her to remain there all night. Instead, she stayed only until the fairgrounds closed nightly. By 6:30 a.m. sharp, she returned again to greet Pilgrim with each new sunrise.

The following month found them at another fair, the Washington Town & Country housed in a much larger venue. After all the showings were over, the auctions began. Ava had known all along that all steers had a final destination; yet, being with Pilgrim for a year and a half had strengthened her bond with him. While the livestock sale at the fair garnered a handsome return, and the "banker" in her relished the investment windfall, turning over the halter and lead rope to an anonymous person led to a tear (or two) that trickled down her cheeks.

"Good-bye, Pilgrim."

The only thing left to do was split the money with her sister Terry. In that regard, Ava negotiated for a more significant cut since it was her time and investment in Pilgrim that won them a substantial check from the sale. Terry countered with her own sound logic: keeping him the extra time had held up her getting any money sooner. The tie-breaker was a 50/50 split.

* * *

Some of Ava's memorable moments as a child harkened back to her early years by way of people whom she and her mom knew, but such shared events also ran throughout her high-school years. One series of incidents reveal another natural side of Ava's diverse interests as she matured.

Sarah's dear friend Sandra, whom she had known since her high-school days, married Gib Fees. The couple lived in the local area, and they had a daughter, Cindy, who was between Ava and Terry in age, and two boys, Syd, a year younger than Ava, and Alex, who was closer to Lanie's age. At first, the Fees children attended a nearby Catholic grade school; graduating to high school, they switched to the public-school system, bringing them into closer contact.

Gib grew up liking fishing and frog catching, and he often went out with his sons. Ava happened to like the older boy, Syd, as much as being out in a boat on a body of water. Whenever Gib came frogging with Syd in tow to the Frick pond, she could be counted on to join the ride.

Frogging, of course, takes place in the dark. Someone steers the boat to the edge of a pond, while another holds a flashlight pointed at the frogs sitting on the bank. The third person is supposed to grab a frog before it jumps back into the water. In the Fees' case, Gib was always the boat driver, and Syd and Ava took turns catching the frogs. As Ava put it, *"OK, mostly Syd snatched the frogs."*

One dark night, the boat was frog heavy. Upon returning to the house, the satisfied trio toted all of the frogs to the basement, where they were left piled on top of each other in a makeshift wire crate. Gib and Syd went upstairs for a moment, and Ava, seeing this mess of live frogs and feeling sorry for them, opened the crate door and let the frogs out. In no time, frogs were hopping all over the place, which did not go over well when Gib returned to the basement. According to Ava, *"Gib was not a happy camper that night!"*

Enter Barbara Heimbaugh, a classmate, and a friend, who in many ways helped develop Ava during her *"growin' up"* years, in particular with watercraft. Ava yearned to drive the boat on some of those frogging nights—in fact, commandeering any floating object would satisfy her itch. Barbara's dad, Ken, was not only the outdoors type but also a patient instructor when it came to teaching canoe skills. He often spent weekends with Barbara and his two boys, Gary and Billy, inviting Ava to come along with them on several occasions. Long-story-short, Ken taught her how to navigate a canoe, which knowledge enabled her to participate in canoe trips down the Bourbeuse River, as well as do raft and inner-tube floating. For Ava, *"... [Those were] exceptional memories."*

Alas, she never did drive the boat on froggin' nights!

Still, animals of all species continued to hold primary interest and positioning in Ava's mind and heart for different reasons, some humorous.

> *"Goats are funny. No way around it. They just are. The kids jump and twist and sail over each other like playing air-born hop-scotch. Goats have a way, when they miscalculate on a jump or antic, of being able to give that look of, "Hey, I meant to do it that way." Recently, it has become fashionable to do what is called Goat Yoga—baby goats climb and jump on the backs of people while they do yoga. This idea comes naturally to goats but is a novel approach for humans to offer up themselves as springboards.*

> *"Back in the early '70s, Six Flags over Mid-America had a 'ride' in the Operations department, sponsored by Purina, called Pet-A-Pet. It had goats, sheep, a calf, pigs (who raced and snorted when chased back to their 'zone'), a fish pond, and, during my tenure there, some exotic deer, a male Llama named Spitz, and a young elephant called Sissy. Even now, I can smell it... a fresh, rural smell. Some of the female goats were nannies, and we milked them during the day, letting kids have a chance at giving it a try. That is until someone decided that touching an*

udder and teats in public was indecent and made us stop.

"On rainy days, the park made available at the front gate some plastic raincoats. I use the word 'coat' loosely. Those were designed to go over clothes and had some kind of a button snap to help keep the wet off garments, but they were made of thin plastic.

"At certain times of the day, we sold grain in cylindrical paper cups for a quarter so people could feed the animals. That became a frenzy of critters, especially the goats, as they got a little age on them, rushing for the grain. Sheep were more polite. The visitors did their best to save some for the special one they had taken a liking to. On those rainy days, there was additional goat fun in store: while one

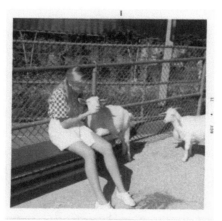

goat was being fed, another would be at the feeder's backside eating this person's

Ava with goats at Pet-a-Pet, Six Flags over Mid-America

*plastic garment about as fast as the grain
was disappearing. By the time the
individual realized there was something
tugging at their backside, it was too late:
they now donned a midriff! We, the
workers at Pet-A-Pet, often laughed that
we were the only ride with a long line
waiting to get out of the turnstile than in!*

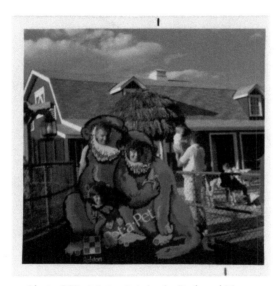

Photo OPP at Pet-a-Pet: Lanie, Dad, and Mom

*"The first goat we owned was an
orphan from this system. The little fella's
mom had been in the herd and was sold;
somehow, he did not go with her. My sister
Phyllis was working at the park at the
time, and someone, knowing she lived on a
farm, enlisted her to come to his aid. He
was fed milk replacer out of a nippled Nehi*

soda bottle. Hence his name, 'Nehi.' Nehi was of the breed called Saanen. For those not familiar with goats, that breed is white, and so was he.

"Life on the farm instantly changed, and many Nehi stories still linger over the land and resurface at family events. He would run into the house if the door was left open too long. He used his best mountain-goat agility to walk along the edge of the truck bed and then marvel at his beauty in the door mirror. Unfortunately, he also itched and Nehi on picnic table *scratched his horns along the side of any tall vehicle left in his traffic lane. One day, when Phyllis came by in her ragtop MG, he took a stroll across the top of it!*

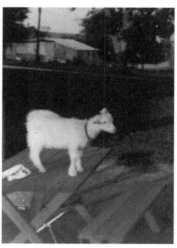

Nehi on a picnic table

Kule/Frick - Conversations with Animals

"I don't remember how old Nehi got to be on the farm because, by then, I was away at college. During an earlier year, Phyllis had acquired a St. Bernard she named Toby, who by now was full grown. She left him at the farm while she was gone, too, and Toby and Nehi became

Nehi looking out the barn loft,

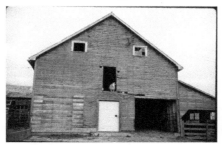

… or, if you prefer, as an adult.

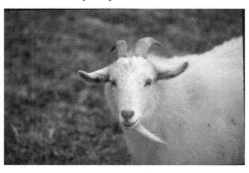

buddies. But, there was a downside to that arrangement.

"Toby had an occasional yearning to take a long walk-about. In the country, that would not have been a problem if he had kept his adventures to the farm. But,

*looking for something else to guard, he
wandered over to the neighbor's acres...
Nehi strolling along for the fun of it with
him. Dad would have to go pick them up.
The sight of Dad driving home with an
oversized St. Bernard and a grown Swiss
goat riding next to him was hilarious. We
sure thought it was funnier than Dad did:
By the third time, he decided enough was
enough, so Nehi took a final ride to the
sale barn."*

* * *

Pre-college activities in the early Seventies were pretty much the same anywhere in America. The Vietnam war was raging, many students called up to serve the country—the most prominent life concern at the time. The draft was in place, making many a guy's goals not his own. In the Bible Belt, America's heartland, emotions ran strong.

*"Family friends and guys from town
were drafted and died in the Vietnam war
during my years of junior high and high
school. The fear of it was everywhere for
loving parents and siblings.*

*"I suppose some of the guys joining
maybe had some feeling of excitement and
patriotism, but most were trying to figure
out how to avoid the conflict and the
dreaded call of their draft number. Our
nation was at odds. The Beatles had been
on the Ed Sullivan Show merely a few
short years earlier, but now serious
Hippies were speaking out."*

Despite the stark influences of jarring, war-time images broadcast into living rooms across the nation through TV news channels, those fortunate enough to remain at home inevitably took on added responsibilities to help around the house, if only to live and grow older day by day. All things considered, despite this, rural farm living remained bucolic.

In Union Missouri, as in other towns and places across the nation, parties where Ava's high-school chums and acquaintances could blow off difficult emotions, steam, and hormones were evening highlights. Ava never participated much in them. For seniors facing college in the fall, impromptu summer parties often materialized in someone's hayfield, and it was not unusual to find among the students a beer keg or two and, rarely, Ava, aside from her high-school graduation celebration.

Tying a ribbon and bow around Alice's horse shows, one must add in loudspeakers mounted on the flatbeds of pickup trucks blaring political messages at parades, a myriad of 4H activities, school bands playing marching music, growing up through changing friendships, seasons, and the inevitable cycles of life and death. With that collage, the picture of Ava's grade- and high-school days and nights at home is completed.

The only place left for her to grow from now on would be away from the farm. Her long-desired college and university years beckoned her on a horizon made of hope. They would include new friendships and lively parties in which Ava participated side-by-side with her peers, though in tiny increments, and mainly when the music featured Jim Croce, The Bee Gees, the Beach Boys, John Denver, and Carole King.

* * *

CHAPTER 4: KNOWING IS POWER

Ava's passion to one day reach out and care for animals was never an easy climb.

"While I certainly acquired a wealth of knowledge growing up, I was never "smart," as my grades reflected. I worked hard to get A's. B's were generally easy, especially B-, but every now and then, I ended up with a C. A's just always stayed a bit out of easy reach. I had to study a lot to get what results I did get. What I have managed to align myself with are common sense, a narrow but deep path of interest, and a degree of vision that gives me unique insights."

Graduation from high school and moving on to higher education at Missouri Valley College (Mo-Val) to study Biology in 1973 was Ava's next step toward her ultimate goal of a university Veterinary College degree. Before that lofty goal could be attained, she would encounter (with blinders firmly in place) events and incidents that could only have happened well beyond Union's city limits. And Marshall, Missouri, was just far enough.

"It was like I had to steal away to be able to 'cut loose.' In some ways, that could make an event all the more exciting;

but, still, as I got into college, I didn't want
to get too attached to any guy for fear a
relationship would get in the way of my
purpose. Nothing was going to stop me
from being a veterinarian ... but I must
say, there was a lot more fun to be had in
college, being away from home for the first
time, and I made the most of it. I was
Treasurer at my Delta Zeta sorority,
College Orientation Chair, and a regular
at the card table in the Sigma Nu, a local
fraternity; perhaps, also, a time or two, to
the detriment of getting to class sober."

Sober or not, Germans do like to party—after all, Oktoberfest offers warm and cold, dark and light beers, plenty of hot 'brats, and fast-paced polkas.

"... But," Ava avowed, *"... my family members were not drinkers. There was no time for that [kind of fun] in my 'Germanville'!"*

Amen.

But, for several farming seasons, Dennis and Owen Frick did grow their own grape crop, and homemade wine did make its way to their tabletops on occasion. Mostly though, the wine provided another way besides hot-water bottles to keep warm during frigid Missouri-winter nights.

Newly enrolled as a collegiate undergrad, Ava made like quite the prankster after she matriculated into Mo-Val, in the process, making a self-discovery.

"There is a mischievous side to me.
This trait runs on Dad's side of the family.
His Uncle Everet, known to everyone as
'Boobley,' was a kidder and fun-loving guy
his entire life ... always up for a prank or

something that would be funny at his expense or others'. So, I believe it just came with the package that I tended to be that way, at times, too. One could say it was in the bloodlines.

"College at Missouri Valley in Marshall presented an excellent opportunity for sorority coeds to do crazy-wild things, and my cohort Diana and I were always up for anything we could imagine.

"One particular winter afternoon, we passed a dead skunk on the road. Brakes on, we turn around, plotting a re-purposing for this deceased skunk.

"Diana had a plastic bag in her trunk that was soon to become the corpse bag.

"We get back to campus and place the bag out by a tree where we were thinkin' nobody would notice it. Alarm set, we arise at 2:00 am to discover three inches of snow on the ground.

"Avoiding extra effort, once the bag is retrieved under a half-moon, we navigate around the potentially incriminating street lights and, the skunk in hand, we make our way to the men's dorm. Stealthily up the stairs we go to the second floor, then down the hallway to the bathroom. There, we deposit the skunk carcass in one of the urinals.

"Manned with a camera to record the deed lest our minds ever failed us, we emblazoned the image on film. But, let it be known that it sure was difficult gettin' out without givin' us up because we were laughin' so hard.

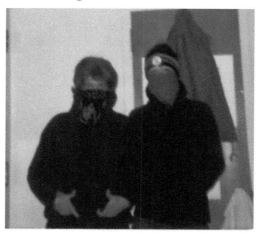

Ava & Diana ready to rumble!

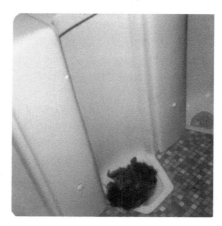

Skunk carcass in urinal

"The next morning at breakfast, a whiff [pun intended] of scuttlebutt about

*something that had happened at the men's
dorm raced through the cafeteria.
Feigning our parts in the dastardly deed,
Diana and I looked as surprised as all the
other girls at our sorority table!*

*"The moral of the story? We got away
with it!*

*"Last year (2018), I attended a Mo-
Val Homecoming, my first one ever, and
'fessed up ... not because of a guilty
conscience—I didn't have one—but
because it was too funny all over again!
And because I could solve their mystery."*

Ava also knew how to take on her male counterparts
inside of their frat house.

*"My skill at card-playing, just like I
took on any game for the victory (too
seriously), landed me in some good Pitch
games at the Sigma Nu fraternity house at
MO-Val. When nine o'clock came, and the
co-eds were supposed to leave the guys'
dorms, I was permitted to stay. Once, a
coed being escorted out asked, 'Why does
she get to stay?' to which a rapid-fire reply
came from one of the guys: 'If you knew
how to play cards as good as she does, you
could stay too...'"*

*"... I'm pretty proud of that. Thanks,
Grandma and Grandpa, for all the hours
of Gin Rummy and Pitch."*

Beyond momentary lettings-off of pent-up steam,
earning the degrees necessary to become a Doctor of

Veterinarian Medicine (D.V.M.) was for years a long-term proposition for Ava, and on a personal level she remained committed to her goal, keeping her extra-curricular activities to a minimum. Yet, from time to time, yearning for her old, familiar comforts, namely her feline companions and other large and small animals, she missed home.

* * *

"Away from home, by my second year in college, I was missing my cats. I guess I had decided there ought to be another in my life, because - I don't remember exactly where she came from – a white kitten with her two irises showing different colors, one blue and one green, appeared. The conundrum was not how she showed up or even why, but what to name her?

(Note: the unusual pairing of those two colors on one cat's eyes is known as 'Waardenburg Syndrome,' which carries a gene for deafness. In this cat's case, the kitten was not born deaf.)

"Since it was 1975, and The Bee Gees were big, a song of theirs aired on my radio. After that, naming her was soon decided: Be for blue and Gee for green.

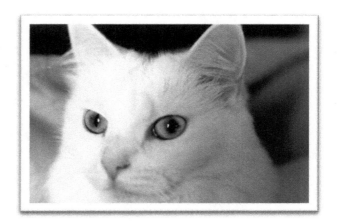

BeGee

"As 'BeGee' grew older, she made a great camping buddy. Together, we took hikes with her wearing a harness. We slept in the tent and toured around in a jeep.

"BeGee protected territories she considered hers. Down in Arizona, no sooner had a sizeable German Shepherd wandered into our yard than, all puffed up, she shot across the yard at that dog. He took off with his tail between his legs. Like a colorful jester absolved of wrongdoing in a king's court, BeGee strutted back across that green lawn proudly. One could almost see the Cheshire grin on her face!

"BeGee lived with me throughout my late teens, twenties, and thirties—a time span of over 19 years. She shared my years of youth when life was full of new experiences, and every day, the beginning of a new adventure. We lived together for

*more years than I lived with my parents
from birth!*

*"Oh, what trouble I would have been
in, though, could she have talked!*

*"To date, I have had no pet with me as
long as that one. Eventually, her kidneys
failed her, and the day came that I knew it
was time to say good-bye. As with so many
days and nights earlier, the final moment
found just the two of us sittin' together. No
one else needed to be there.*

*"BeGee loved to sit off the east porch
of the clinic in Union and gaze at her
realm, which, to me, seemed to be the one
right place to rest her ashes, and so I did."*

* *

Beyond study, and wanting to participate in formal extra-curriculars at Marshall, Ava played flute in the band, ran track, took Weight-Training classes—her first introduction to learning about how to work muscles, and gained membership into the national biology fraternity, Beta Beta Beta (BBB). In 1976, seasoned and ready to expand her horizon closer to her goal, she transferred to the grossly larger main campus and student body of the University of Missouri in Columbia; specifically, to their College of Veterinary Medicine.

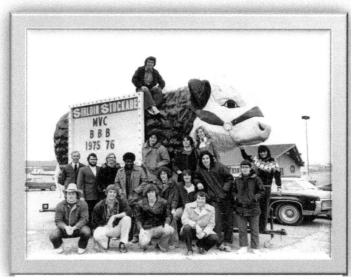

Missouri Valley College Beta Beta Beta Biology Fraternity

One recalls that there were no computers, cell phones, smartphones, or PowerPoint presentations back then. Just books and professors; notebooks, pens, pencils, overhead projectors, carousel slides … and lively, real conversations with class and dorm mates.

An Animal Science major there, who had known briefly of Ava from earlier school days, commented, "Ava and I shared some of the classes in common. I could see that she was adjusting to the change from attending classes with eight to 10 students in attendance to the university's norm of about 500 attendees. She kinda had that 'deer in the headlights' look about her in the earliest days of her university residency but, being bright, smart, and intelligent, she adapted quickly, even though she didn't appear to live on-campus. Once I remembered she was from where I came from, I realized it was possible that during breaks, she still may live at home in Union near where I had grown up."

Ava more than adapted to the big campus. She rode her bike to class, weather permitting—a distance of 1.7 miles—and, when taking breaks from study, picked up her flute or jogged for exercise. She even learned to play Bridge in the lounge with other students between classes!

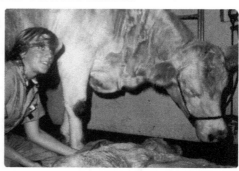

Ava with cow & calf delivered in veterinary college

Because of skills learned early on, Ava enjoyed certain advantages and was ahead of her classmates in the application side of her chosen field, but not so when it came to theory study. Her academic journey was *"... plain not easy"* for her. Only with help from friends and a paid (in cookies) tutor, plus her own hard work over many hours cracking the books, would she make it all the way. Relief from those pressures came to her by driving to and from visits to her family or to visit a sister while listening to Willie Nelson songs ("Mamas Don't Let Your Babies Grow Up to Be Cowboys"), or singing the Roy Rogers' anthem, "Happy Trails."

Other times, she re-discovered her lightheartedness with regular visits and time spent visiting with the generous Irishman she had met in her teenaged years. By now, Dr. McGinity was her Large Animal Medicine and Surgery professor and, of course, she happily occupied a place within his heart, having fulfilled her promise to return as one of his students.

Among her peers and other professors, it wasn't a secret that Ava struggled with certain aspects of her Veterinary studies; some parts were downright tricky for her to grasp or memorize. Dr. McGinity to the rescue: he was always there for her if she needed to ask questions or have him simply listen and offer advice. The kindly man always answered her questions as best he could, even a philosophical one that was a rather tall order, even in her eyes, *"How do you know what's important enough to get upset about and when to let it go?"*

McGinity's simple and profound answer floored his inquisitive student: "I always ask myself, *'In 100 years, is it going to matter?'"*

His answer became not only a guiding light for Ava but also a datum that calmed her down whenever her anxieties tried to take control. She now had a way to be self-sufficient in the face of any problem demanding a decision that would affect her future existence and those of the animals she would meet. In short, McGinity was Ava's go-to person of choice and her designated V.I.P. (Very Important Person).

McGinity continued to have a calming effect upon Dr. Frick as the years slipped by and his time on Earth pressed onward. By the time, many years later, she received a phone call from his daughter, Ann, giving her the news that her father was on his way out—"Ava, I knew you would want to know," Ava already had carved out a cherished place in her heart for his kindnesses, wisdom, and gentle manner with her.

(NOTE: In 1970, Dr. Joseph T. McGinity received the Norden Distinguished Teaching Award. In his 22 years as a faculty member teaching Large Animal Medicine and Surgery, he achieved statewide and national recognition for his expertise in the field. He also earned recognition from the Veterinary Medical Alumni Association and was awarded the UMC Alumni Association Award of Merit given annually to an outstanding alumnus of the college.)

Whenever *If I can just get to the practical application ... get to the clinics, then I know I can make it* ran through Ava's mind, the good Irish doctor/professor's helpful words and manner assisted her through her study challenges.

Also, her grandma's teaching.

> *"[Because of my sewing with grandma], I was way ahead of most in the surgery class, especially the guys, who had never picked up a needle before! When I had the broken arm in the 4th grade, I learned to do things with my left hand, and after spending that time learning to be quasi left-handed, I was determined to keep some of that skill. It paid off because being somewhat ambidextrous in surgery was advantageous, to say the least."*

* * *

Ava's sister Lanie expressed gratitude for the skillful attention her sister gave to her during a rough time after her pet dog had her leg broken when Dennis ran over it with his tractor. Ava gladly came to her little sister's rescue.

> *"An incident happened while I was in vet school. Jenny Rebecca, my sister Lanie's collie dog, was brought in after she had been hit because I was in the college, and the injuries were more than the local vet felt comfortable tackling. I was in a different rotation and had not done either the anesthesia or surgery block, but they let me come in to assist/observe. Unfortunately, the sterile room and chemical-antiseptic smells, and crunching on the leg of the dog, all got to*

me. I remember asking Lloyd Kloppe, the student monitoring anesthesia, if he thought it was hot in there.

"About the third time I had that thought, I fainted into the surgeon and hit the floor, coming to only after a Vet Tech (assistant technician) had propped me up against the wall. The surgery did go well, and Jenny was allowed to go home with Lanie and Dad a few days later.

"This was actually the second time I got faint in a vet clinic; the first was back in Marshall during a surgery. The anesthetic smells had been too much, but I was able to leave the room for some fresh air before I passed out."

For Lanie's dog, that break required major orthopedic surgery. When she re-broke the leg a second time, Ava searched in vain for ways to fix it for her saddened, 14-year-old sister. This time, forced to inform Lanie that the leg should be amputated and that its loss would significantly impair the quality of living for the rest of the dog's life, she employed a quiet, professional manner. She assisted Lanie by

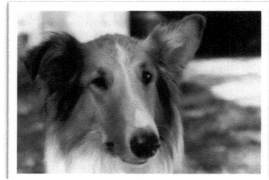

Jenny Rebecca

explaining her options, which included putting the pet down, and helped her face the horrendously tricky situation.

*"I was still in vet school when Jenny
got hit the second time. I must have come
home for the weekend to help her decide."*

The two sisters often had observed many animal births and deaths together. To them, such options had matured to merely a fact of farm life. Still, this one hit close to home for them. In the end, Lanie felt grateful that her older sister had presented only options without any attempt to persuade her one way or the other. She asked Ava to transport Jenny to another veterinarian to be euthanized there.

Reflecting and, perhaps, trying to find some levity to change the way she felt then, and still feels today about the incident, Lanie recalled that she had thought something incongruous at the time: Garrison Keillor of *A Prairie Home Companion* had said on his radio show, "Cats were considered royalty in Egyptian times and they never have forgotten that."

Odd at the time, the thought had made her smile throughout the profound quiet following her decision to let her cherished pet dog be put down.

* * *

Outside of Ava's busy curriculum schedule, time to blow off the buildup of emotions and data rattling in her head was rare, but for her, a bit of dancing never hurt. Disco was the rage in the later years of the 1970s, and occasionally she was right there on the dance floor of a local studio, learning the latest steps to the musical soundtrack of *Saturday Night Fever* with partners from all corners. One such evening added a plot-point twist to her life that she never saw coming.

Ava always wanted to take a disco dance lesson, and she found a local community center offering lessons. Having signed up, she cajoled a vet-school classmate to partner with her.

> *"It was the fall of 1978. I begged*
> *Lanny Weddle, a classmate, to be my*
> *Disco dance partner for some community*
> *classes. The first night, he skipped class*
> *for a greater priority: the World Series.*
> *So, there I was without a partner, but not*
> *for long. There was another young*
> *partner-less student, so it kind of worked*
> *out between us that he, Bill Johnson, a*
> *Med student, and me, a Veterinarian-to-be,*
> *danced all night. In September 1979, we*
> *married."*

* * *

Ava's seven years of collegiate studies through 1980 ended with an unexpected reward in her senior year: the A.H. Growth Student Research Award presented to her by Professor Corwin in recognition of her senior year's stellar work in parasitology (the study of parasitic organisms). With that, it appeared the Universe finally returned the favor for all her newly, hard-won knowledge and extended hours of study and application at home and inside classrooms. Not long after, her most-cherished dream came true the day she clutched her long-coveted Doctor of Veterinary Medicine diploma in her hand.

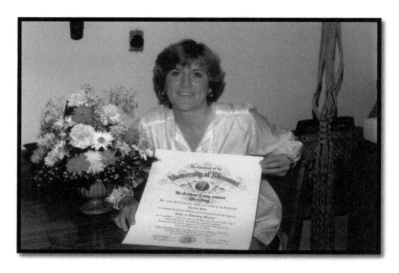

Ava with diploma

She and the other 69 students of her close-knit, graduating class could commence their careers after professing their loyalty to the Veterinarian Oath.

"Being admitted to the profession of veterinary medicine, I solemnly swear to use my scientific knowledge and skills for the benefit of society through the protection of animal health and welfare, the prevention and relief of animal suffering, the conservation of animal resources, the promotion of public health, and the advancement of medical knowledge.

"I will practice my profession conscientiously, with dignity, and in

keeping with the principles of veterinary medical ethics.

"I accept as a lifelong obligation, the continual improvement of my professional knowledge and competence."

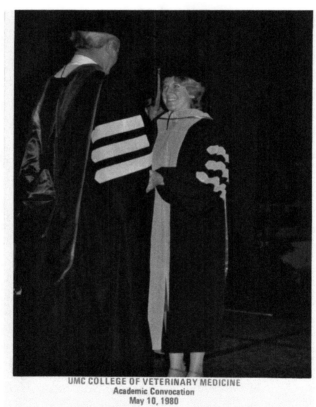

UMC COLLEGE OF VETERINARY MEDICINE
Academic Convocation
May 10, 1980

Graduation ceremony with Dean Corley

"Seven to eight years of college from the front side looks like 'forever,' but from

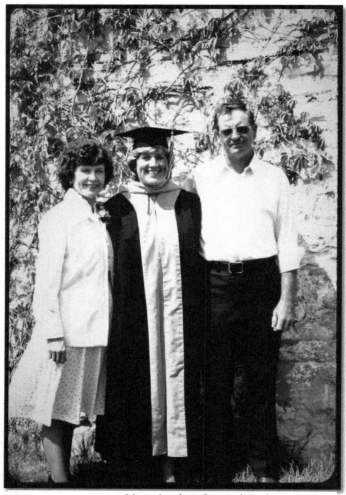

Mom, Ava (cap & gown), Dad

*the rear-view mirror, that was a moment in
time that had passed all too soon. Those
were some of the best years of my life ...
and collection of the best friends to boot!"*

Classmates at reunion. Lanny Weddle, 2nd from left

Many from the same graduating class would continue to share their journey and remain in touch. They re-convene every five years like clockwork at scheduled reunions.

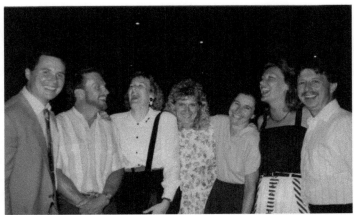

Classmates reunion. Danny Weddle 2nd from left.

* * *

With her college days behind her, the magnitude of the horizon ahead of her and her primary purpose in her estimation changed Ava's behavior patterns for the better:

> *"Once ordained as a Doctor of*
> *Veterinarian Medicine, having taken THE*
> *oath and promised to 'above all do no*
> *harm,' my focus and responsibility level*
> *rose. My inclination to cut loose and be*
> *funny or silly declined while I was on duty,*
> *which bled over to life at home…"*

* * *

Merely a year later, Ava's husband graduated from Med school in 1981. The couple's marriage was merely a year and a half old at this point. In the intervening months, they lived a split life mostly between Columbia, Missouri, and Mission, Kansas—scores of miles separate the two towns. When possible, they shared the mutually satisfying activities of photography, bicycling, and playing musical instruments—he, the accordion, and she, of course, flute.

Symbiotes of science, Doctors Ava Lee Frick, D.V.M., and William Lee Johnson, M.D., were also, however, products of the two different lifestyles they knew growing up. His city-bred life ade him used to living among crowds of people in tight spaces; hers was all about animals and wide-open-spaces country living. With Dr. Johnson working to complete his time in school and earn his M.D. from Columbia, Dr. Frick forged ahead by working in her new career in another town. The distance and days and nights apart afforded each ample space to consider honestly what their future together might be like, as Ava observed wryly, *"The funny thing was that we never made dancing a regular event after we finished our first Disco dance lessons."*

* * *

CHAPTER 5: JAM-PACKED '80s

Dr. Frick sailed into the practical side of her career right after graduation, ending up at a rural mixed-animal practice in Richland, Missouri, for a few months. The second weekend after she was on duty, the practice owners Dr. Max Thornsberry and his wife Brenda, having the opportunity of another doctor on board, took some sorely needed time off and left the new doctor alone to run their clinic by herself for better or worse.

Early one Saturday morning, the emergency line rang loudly. A man calling said they had a cow about to calve. They had felt three legs but not a fourth. The caller explained that they usually did not call someone in at this stage, but they felt this time that they wanted a doctor out with them.

Dr. Frick, the only one on duty at the time, was "It."

When she arrived at the family farm, the man she spoke with earlier informed his visitor that the cow in question was actually their favorite "pet." Somehow, the cow got mixed up with their bull—an act they never intended to happen.

Straight away, he led Dr. Frick to a wooded area where the cow was in labor. She observed that it was a reasonably clean spot, so whatever had to happen, if needed, could be done right there. Gloved up, she began a palpation examination of the cow. Reaching in vaginally, she felt for legs, counting one... two... three... four... FIVE! That told her there were twins in there!

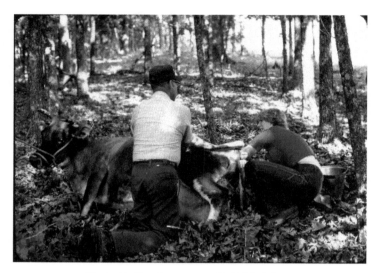

Mr. Ledbetter, Jersey cow, Dr. Frick doing exam

Not wanting to bring these twin calves out piece by piece, a C-section seemed the best approach to Dr. Frick. She reminded herself that even though she only recently graduated with her degree, she probably could pull this off successfully.

Right about then, the cow's owner Harvey Ledbetter, stepped up, rubbed his stubbled chin, and asked a simple, leading question, "I guess you have done these before?"

"Yes, we did them in the large-animal block," bluffed Frick, referring to surgeries she had *observed* in veterinary college.

> *"There were no cell phones back then.*
> *No way to dial in Dr. Thornsberry for*
> *guidance. It was all up to me to consider*
> *what I knew, what I thought I knew, and*
> *then do it."*

"Well, do I have time to go get 'Mother' here? She had a caesarian with two of our kids, I think she may want to watch," added Ledbetter. He turned and walked toward the house. Frick answered almost under her breath in a whisper, *"Sure, you do."*

Frick quickly prepped the cow for the C-section. She wanted to get both calves out of her in the shortest time possible. The surgery proved partially successful—she saved the mother cow, but both calves were still-born.

No shouts of joy sprang from the onlooking bystanders; no congratulations to the doctor for her work. The owners did thank her. Frick knew there was a small victory in the fact that the favorite, the 12-year-old pet cow survived.

The thought that she had just experienced her first open-field surgery much in the manner that James Herriot wrote about it in his book *All Creatures Great and Small,* comforted Dr. Frick. Though the event was a pyrrhic victory and a trial under fire with mixed results, she accomplished what she must the best she knew how.

Real living is visceral. There is birth, continuance, death … and rebirth. To really feel alive, we must, each of us, find and strike a balance between life and death, embracing all.

This is what I was put here on Earth to do loudly rang between Frick's ears on her return to the clinic. Feeling humbled, awed, and tired, yet sated, she knew in her heart and mind that the whole seven-plus years of toil and struggle for the knowledge and skills she now possessed were all worth it!

As profound as the overall event was, the technique Frick employed to make her discovery of the twins served as hard evidence to citified laypersons. What they might consider an unworthy task—introducing a gloved hand and arm into a bovine vagina or rectum to feel for what one is looking to find ("palpation")—and might be considered crude to the uninitiated, is, in fact, a standard practice. Even though it may yield successful or disheartening results that affect profoundly animal owners and veterinarian doctors alike, science rests on its application when necessary. On the other hand, not everything about Veterinarian Medicine is as severe regarding rectal matters.

> *"Sunday dinner after church in the*
> *Ozarks meant fried chicken, mashed*
> *potatoes, gravy, and green beans. Another*
> *routine of the Lord's Day was to give the*
> *leftover chicken bones to the dogs. Now,*
> *while they were tasty going down, too*
> *many poultry bones, being porous, are*
> *quite constipating. By Thursday, calls to*
> *the clinic inevitably started coming in*
> *about dogs straining to defecate. So, out*
> *came the enema bags; on some days for as*
> *many as three dogs waiting their turn.*
> *Thursdays, therefore, came to be known*
> *around the clinic as 'Enema Day.'"*

* * *

Shortly after her summer run in Richland, Dr. Frick moved to Kansas City, intent on working under the tutelage of Dr. James Guglielmino for a year. The animal hospital system there had a central hospital and several satellite clinics, one of which, in Overland Park Kansas, Dr. Frick would run, sending all surgeries to be performed at the central hospital in Mission, Kansas. Animals picked up via a shuttle left more time for her to put in work and gain valuable experience at the clinic or the main hospital.

Dr. Guglielmino recalled: "I do remember that Dr. Frick was married to an M.D. at the time because when I interviewed her, I was a bit put off by the fact that he had come to our town with her; it led me to wonder if she was her own person. However, that concern was quickly put away because he did not stay, and it became apparent to me that Dr. Frick was a very independent person. Her duties and responsibilities were all the duties and responsibilities of a practicing small-animal veterinarian, which included both medicine and surgery."

While the idea of being an "everything" doctor to all animals fit with her farm-life resumé, over time Frick realized that her skills were best applied to small animals: mostly cats and dogs without eliminating "pocket" pets— hamsters, for example, are among the tiniest of living creatures.

"One day, a family came to the clinic, composed of both parents, two girls eight and six years old, and their two pet hamsters, each in its own rolly ball. The oldest daughter's hamster was alright, but the younger child's pet had a sizeable mammary tumor. The lifespan of a hamster is around two to three years, and they are very inexpensive pocket pets; yet, neither of those points were pertinent to the girls' parents. Instead, they were about teaching their girls that every life has value; that no matter what side of the street you come from or how poor or small you may appear, the wealth of one's experience is not what's essential; life itself is.

"I could see the hesitation in the younger girl's eyes as she handed me her hamster, and I knew what she was feeling, what she feared. Discussing with the family what it would cost and what could be the possible worst and best scenarios, I assured them that I would do my very best

*to make sure that the hamster would go
home later that day, without guarantee.
The young girl petted her little friend and
kissed her on the head, hoping it would not
be the last time.*

*"The surgery went well. The hamster
returned home with the family to play in
her rolly ball again.*

*"I think back, now and then, at how
differently those two young girls may have
grown up and looked at life had their
parents been selfish and short-sighted. And
for me, this was more than saving the
hamster. This was a living, breathing
example of ethics, morals, and cultural
value sustained for every living creature,
no matter how small."*

* * *

Soon after Bill Johnson's graduation from medical school, the professionally sanctioned couple headed to Phoenix, Arizona, where he would do his Pediatrics internship. Departing Kansas in their CJ 7 Jeep with only bare necessities packed for the trip, BeGee along for the ride, and no job position lined up for Frick, the adventure felt to them like a fresh start. Upon arrival, the couple met up with Frick's classmate Lloyd Kloppe and his wife, Jana. At least for the first leg of their Southwest stint, they would share their place.

With only two priorities in mind—finding a permanent place to live and a job of her own, Dr. Frick wasted no time accomplishing her goals. She took a position at the Arizona Humane Society (AzHS), feeling good that she had landed a great job with a better-than-average pay rate at $15.00 per hour.

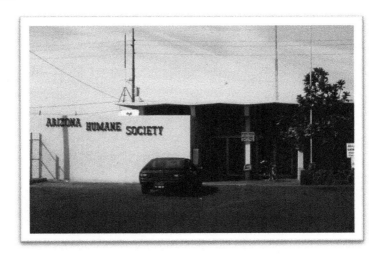

Arizona Humane Society, 1981

Another newly graduated veterinarian, Dr. Jim Prater, who worked at the same place, quickly made himself known to Frick. Long hours spent putting in hard work at the AzHS (whose veterinary hospital split off within two years of her arrival to become the Dubois Memorial Veterinary Hospital) enabled a friendly relationship to arise from the sheer proximity of two peer-level veterinarians working under the same roof. Beyond the usual surgeries, medical cases, and administrative duties, writing their reports often placed them in the same room for long stretches of time.

Eschewing the formality of their earned titles, Prater invited Ava and Bill (despite his more often staying on-duty at the hospital where he worked) to a number of parties at his house. One, he recalled, was a daytime get-together over BBQ and the backyard swimming pool. The friendly outing moved from ordinary to legendary the moment Ava and another BBQ attendee took up a dare to jump from the house rooftop into the deep end of the chlorinated backyard pool!

They made quite a splash among the guests (pun intended) and left Prater with a mental picture that, to this day, owns an indelible piece of real estate in his mind. He cannot remember, however, if she held her nose or not—she contends she did not—as she flew through the air.

Prater, laughing, also recalled another stunt that Frick performed that same day—one he never saw anyone do before. Bouncing on the edge of the diving board, she suddenly threw her legs out in front of her and let her bottom slap the board's end on the downbeat, bouncing her up into the air, from where she pitched forward straight into the pool. "Ham and Eggs" (as it was called) was a stunt she had learned at school parties. With no Olympic judges present to score her form, the party-goers applauded and laughed along with her for having the courage to do the stunt.

> *"Generally, no drinking was done at home during the week, but parties were a different story. I would partake if they were playing Boy George, Cyndi Lauper, U2, or Prince on the stereo speakers ... hey, it was the Eighties!"*

Despite party antics and her loud plays of then-popular songs—Cindy Lauper's "Girls Just Wanna Have Fun", Boy George's "Chameleon;" U2, George Strait, Elton John, and George Jones, an eclectic mix, for sure, the news of the times surrounding Frick and friends was not all fun and games: Close-by, south of the Arizona border, thousands died in southern Mexico the day the volcano El Chichón erupted; Tylenol capsules laced with potassium cyanide killed seven in Chicago and scared millions; screen-legend Princess Grace Kelly died in a fatal car crash, and major recession hit the United States.

Getting back to the grindstone of making a living was going to be tough. After all, veterinary medicine is not as natural as it might appear to a layperson. After nearly 10 years of rigorous study and classroom lab work, many burnings of the midnight oil, and pulling all-nighters at home, Dr. Frick earned her distinguished diploma and credentials but had traded them for the limited privilege of wrestling with, and getting bitten or clawed by, animals of all shapes, sizes, and breeds.

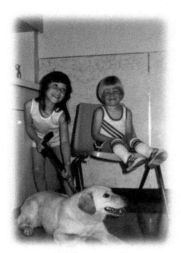

two kids happy to have a new friend, Sandy

Despite these downsides, Dr. Frick's windshield and rear-view mirror recognized no other way of life or living as more worthy or satisfying than working with the animals under her care.

Dr. Prater commented, "There were shifting sands surrounding the thin borderline of communication and responsibility between a Veterinarian and the patient's owners."

Looking back at Dr. Frick's work there, he estimated her acuity with animals against her requirements for blowing off steam:

"Dr. Frick, I know, is a top-notch Veterinarian. Back when we worked in the same clinic, she worked hard. She partied hard, too. We were young then—fresh out of Vet school. We were socially active. I remember at least one time that she showed up at my house wearing a house mouse Halloween costume to our October party.

"Yep, she was a hard worker who also could hang loose away from the clinic. Her bottom line, though, was that she loved animals her whole life and all of the time. We both did, in fact, and we both have our share of scars from the times we took bites for the Cause!"

Prater further contributed his insights about a strange phenomenon he had observed about veterinary candidates at the time, "Three-fourths of women pursuing this career knew all of their years that this is what they wanted to do when they grew up. Among men, the percentage is way down from there. Perhaps, there is an emotional attachment for women; and a logical, factual, pragmatic leaning inside of men?"

For sure, Dr. Frick knew that she wanted to work with animals and provide their healthcare since she was three. Prater's becoming a Veterinarian, on the other hand, was a matter of his not-knowing until after his second year of college what career to choose. He took an aptitude-and-interests test and found "Veterinary Medicine" at the top of his recommended list of occupations. With a shrug and a smile, he decided, "… that was as good as any career to get into for life."

Equally not as surprising is that Dr. Prater's approach to the practice of the profession aligned more with the decided majority percentage of certified veterinarians who express themselves as followers of a "Western" approach to healthcare, which searches for the underlying general cause of an illness or problem and removes that cause. (Example: When an animal has a swollen foot from a burr attached to it, one removes the burr.)

According to Prater, coming from the other gender or not, Dr. Frick operated more intuitively toward each individual animal she treated. At one time, however, she discovered her intuition not as finely tuned as it should have been.

"When I worked at the Arizona Humane Society on Dunlap, there was a boarding place across the street called Doggie Dude Ranch. They had a pet tarantula named Elvira. (Yes, a spider, an arachnid, but a pet nonetheless.)

"One day, Dee, one of the ranch hands, came over to tell me Elvira was acting weird. I strolled over to take a look-see ... not that I was any tarantula expert. But I was not opposed to spiders, including this one which would crawl on my arms, now and then.

"(Yeah, a little creepy, but safe.)

"Right away, looking her over, I see fleas. The resident, long-haired, fluffy cat, who slept on top of her terrarium, was discovered on closer inspection to be the source of Elvira's infestation.

"Now, what to do about it?

"I instructed Dee to take a cotton ball and put very little of a water-based pyrethrin spray on it. Then dab the fleas and pick them off.

"BIG MISTAKE!

"At that moment in time, I had thought of Elvira as a furry pet, not a spider that

*succumbs to insect killers containing
pyrethrins. Nothing had hit me about this
fact and my suggestion. I had been guilty
of looking at Elvira too much like a pet
and not, as others might, a spider to be
crushed out of its existence as fast as
possible.*

*"The next day, I was told that Elvira
is dead. Only then did it hit me: 'OMG! I
killed Elvira! I felt terrible.'*

*"I had to take more responsibility
than just saying I was sorry, so I went out
and bought another 'Elvira,' though not
the Elvira we all knew and loved.*

* * *

Life in her humane-society environment had happy
moments, too, like when an old dog got a great second home,
a little boy got his first puppy, or a lost pet returned to its
loving family.

*"Back then, when we needed a blood
transfusion for an animal at the clinic, we
could go pick one at the shelter to donate.
We would look for one who had been there
a while and repeatedly had been
overlooked, even though it was a
wonderful dog or cat. After the blood
donor's contribution had been completed,
it would rest at the hospital for a day
before we returned the animal to the
shelter with a big cage sign announcing
that he or she had donated blood to save
another animal's life, adding that all
he/she needed now was a loving home: A*

*righteous plea of 'Please Adopt Me! I gave
blood to save another dog's life.'"*

* * *

However, reflecting life on this planet, not every clinical
experience begins with an uplifting start or ends with a
happy outcome. There always is plenty of work to be done,
some of it hazardous to extremes not easily imagined.

In mid-1985, a giant Husky, which Dr. Frick attempted
to help, bit into her severely. Dr. Prater heard about it almost
as soon as it happened. Unfortunately, he never saw the
incident in real-time, because veterinarians seldom share the
same rooms when operating on or handling a patient. He did
hear that she accepted the event stoically as part of her
passion and career. He was told that she also had been, after
the incident, adamant about the owners thinking twice before
taking the dog home. They disagreed and took the
unpredictable and unstable dog to a house in which small
children lived, angering Frick considerably.

*"That was the first time in my life I
ever needed surgery. [From the start], the
dog was angry-looking and growled, so he
had been muzzled. As I removed the muzzle
at the completion of the standard wellness
exam, I was looking at the owner and
talking to him about the demeanor of this
dog. The split second that clip was
loosened on the muzzle, he swung around
and had my left arm in his mouth. The
gnawing of his teeth through the muscle of
my arm sent me screaming. By the third
chomp, the guy grabbed at the rear end of
the dog. The canine let loose of me and
wheeled around to nab his next victim.
(The "new" owner swore this was the*

same dog they had kept three years earlier, which had been taken from them.)

"Maybe in body but certainly not in mind *was my thought.*

"With my arm freed, I quickly exited the room and headed to the sink across the hall. The second I shook my arm, muscle tissue plastered my pant leg and sink. The technicians present rallied quickly, and Nancy Duffield took me to the hospital down the street. Within 90 minutes, I had received an examination, the wound was cultured—24 hours later, nine different bacteria had grown up—and an IV catheter was in place. A surgeon who specialized in arm surgeries was en route to perform the initial surgery that night. A second one came the next day, followed by three days in the hospital under observation before I headed home for two weeks on IV antibiotics. Only then could I return to work at least partial hours in the clinic..."

An athlete, Frick was anxious to get back in the "game."

"... My rehabilitation consumed a large part of the next five months of my life and, believe it or not, it was my first exposure to physical therapy (PT), setting an interest for me to know more about it as a subject as well as a useful tool for animals.

"Total function eventually returned, but the deep scars are still there on both

sides of my left arm—reminders of a point in time of this life of mine and the lesson that changed forever how I would handle aggressive dogs."

* * *

Some vet experiences were so heartbreaking they would try anybody's soul, including Dr. Frick's, to find the virtue of forgiveness in one's heart … or a dry eye and a Kleenex.

"My heart still aches when I remember this: I worked for six years at the Arizona Humane Society. As at any shelter, the employees there had seen many unbelievable cases of abuse wreaked upon innocent animals, but this day a woman brought us a roughly nine-week-old kitten—roughly estimated because the poor thing was undernourished, making his head appear a little bit out of proportion to the rest of his body. The woman had taken him from a couple of boys she had determined to be 10 or 12 years old, who had cigarette lighters in their hands; they had been burning the kitten with the flame from those lighters.

"I set aside my emotions and got to work, taking the kitten in my hand, and beginning the assessment. His tiny ears were burned, as were his whiskers now curled up, no longer the long feelers they had been. The fur on his legs was soot-blackened from the spot of the flame. His little scrotum was burned and now red, raw, and furless.

"I got some gentle soap and put his tiny body into a sink (with a towel placed on the bottom for his comfort), intending to give him a bath and try to help soothe his wounds. As I ran the water and gently lathered him up, he looked up at me with big eyes. Meowing loudly, he began to purr. By this time, I had tears in my eyes, because the very image of what an hour ago had been inflicting pain on him [a human], he seemed now so willing to forgive.

"How could this be? No grudge, no getting even, no hate, no blame. Am I staring at a perspective of life that includes being right in the moment? Is this what true forgiveness is all about? *my thoughts both tore at me and uplifted me.* This moment in his short life, for him, is right. He has forgotten and (seemingly) forgiven.

"We got him healed and fed, and, when he was ready to be adopted, we wrote up his story and hung it on his cage. Soon, a line of people wanting to show him that not all humans are wrong and that there would be a beautiful life ahead for him had gathered."

* * *

Moved by the memory of that abused kitten and its will to forgive despite the horrors faced at the hands of those boys, Dr. Frick remembered another event that involved the *caring* attitude of another pet's owners, and what that feeling did for them as a couple:

"I remember this older couple who came to the DuBois Memorial Hospital at the Arizona Humane Society. Their dog had a lung tumor and needed a lobectomy (surgical removal of that lung lobe). The morning that they left him for the radiographs and blood tests, the wife was crying. She was afraid they didn't have the money it would take to save him.

"Her husband gently patted her hand and said, 'It will be ok, Honey, I have some money saved.'

"Realistically, in her sorrow, I don't think she grasped the full extent of what he was saying.

"As their story unfolded, on their return to pick him up after his successful surgery, Poppa, I found out, had been stockpiling cash in a hidden jar for years in the event of an emergency! And here was the perfect time to bring the pot out and dig into it a bit.

"My heart was touched, reminded that 'Where Love abounds, all things are possible.'"

* * *

Yes, although fully trained in Western-style Veterinary Medicine, after years of experiences like these, Dr. Frick's intuition and skills moved her to explore and add to her arsenal of care other modalities of diagnosis and treatment, which she would use for the greater good (and personal benefit) of each animal that came her way. In her growth, she aligned herself with both schools of the medical arts: the allopathic, which suppresses symptoms while getting at the cause; and the less rigorous homeopathic, which parallels natural body function by treating symptoms with a "like-treats-like" approach. (For example, a rash can be treated by applying another controlled "rash," triggering the body's natural defenses to handle the outbreak, regardless of the cause.) In other words, Western medicine assumes a body needs outside help, i.e., drugs, while the other understands the body can use a similar stimulus to help marshal its own forces to correct a non-optimum situation.

Both Doctors Prater and Frick continued to work as veterinarians in the approach they felt was right for them. Research among the ranks of their respective peers continued to evolve and expand boundaries of known data across several related sciences that could contribute to Veterinary Medicine. Frick learned more and more beyond the scope of the static, old-school approach of her respected peer and friend. They both did good work; they each respected the other's prerogatives.

* * *

Three more years passed, and Dr. Johnson completed his residency in Pediatric Internal Medicine. In their time together in Arizona, Ava and he found a number of differences between them, most notably their job requirements. His schedule placed him on-call all the time, 24/7; hers allowed for free weekends. All too often, they ended up under the same roof but running two different lives on two different levels—not the best recipe for a healthy, long-lasting marriage.

By 1984, Frick decided to cast herself adrift from her relationship with Johnson. He moved back to Missouri and took a specialty position there. She remained in Arizona for another three years.

Upon his retirement, her old friend and professor, Dr. McGinity, took several Elder Hostel trips to Arizona. Inevitably, he ended up jaunting up to Phoenix to visit with his former student. A welcome guest anytime, he uplifted her spirits with his sense of humor and his fondness for her.

For her part, knowing by then exciting places to go in the area, Frick shared with McGinity popular spots where interactive entertainment might be on tap. In particular, she took him to a place where a chicken played Tic-tac-toe with customers willing to ante up at 25 cents a pop to try to beat the hen! Here's how it worked: The participant would pay in his/her quarter-dollar, and the bird would come out through a trap door and make the first move on the game board, inevitably winning the game. A win for the hen meant another trap door would open, and she would be rewarded with some corn.

Standing in front of her former professor and desperately wanting to impress him, the 26-year-old Dr. Frick vied against the bird for the win at least five or six (losing) times. McGinity, every time, howled with laughter at her efforts, not so much because she lost but because of how frustrated she got at the "unfortunate" outcomes! For many a visit later, he still howled over his recall of the veterinarian he'd taught, who simply could not beat a chicken! And, because he also knew how much she was a doggedly persistent student of the science they shared a love for, as well as a gifted one, made the recall all the more hilarious, if not precious, to him. Until his passing several years later, the two remained special friends.

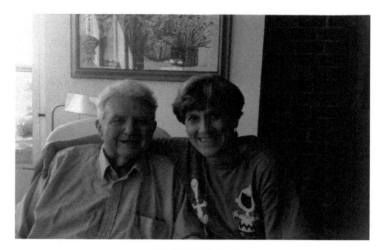

Dr. McGinity & Ava

* * *

Single, willing to try new things and be good at all of them, Frick got the notion that snow skiing was a challenge she should master in the winter of 1985. Having decided one day to drive to Flagstaff to get in some practice—a drive that entailed several hours on the highway from Phoenix and more coming back home, she had it in her mind to go and do this no matter what anyone else thought, despite no one else available to go with her. With her mind made up, she took off.

Up to now, her experience on skis had been minimal. Snow gear and skis on, she rode the lift to the top of the slope, where the sheer steepness, combined with the previous day's warmer temperatures and last night's freezing left the white surface as slick as glass. Undaunted, she lowered her goggles, took a deep breath, and pushed off. After only a few feet, she found herself speeding toward the woods. She snowplowed to slow down, but the breaking maneuver was not working. A split-second later, she fell to her right. Her left leg still adorned with a long ski, hit the ground, flew up in full extension, and slammed down again with a horrible crunch. She damaged her left knee, but the only way to end this nightmarish, lonely incident was to somehow get down the hill. What came next was not pretty.

Passing perilously close by other skiers, tears from the pain streaking icicles onto her nearly frozen cheeks, she hollered for people to look out as she flew downhill at break-neck speed until somehow she landed in a giant snowdrift piled up by the grooming machine operator at the base of the hill.

Injured, embarrassed, and nursing a rapidly swelling left knee that throbbed with pain, she drove the long distance home.

Diagnosis the next day revealed severely stretched medial and lateral collateral knee ligaments. Bandaged up and on crutches, she lay low for a while.

Simultaneously, other changes took place, some about to hit Dr. Frick's pathway. Dr. Chris Snodgrass had purchased the Dubois Memorial Veterinary Hospital, moved the business to 7th Street, and re-named it Mountain View Animal Hospital (MVAH). He hired Dr. Frick to go work with him. Now she would work for the very man whom she met while working at the Marshall Animal Clinic years earlier. Serendipity came along in the person of someone who would become a lifelong friend: Nancy McCafferty, a letter carrier for the USPS, who delivered mail to a list of route customers that included MVAH.

Coming and going as she did for her work, McCafferty noticed that the "tan-colored-like-Arizona" clinic located in a recently developed strip-mall was always clean and modern. She saw that the staff seemed to meet and treat their customers with warm welcomings. After a few cordial conversations in passing through, she and Dr. Frick became fast friends. Frick, in fact, began visiting McCafferty's house with some regularity.

McCafferty, too, felt she now had a new friend.

"I had liked her from the beginning because I could see she was well-respected for her business ethics and that she was a good doctor. She looked at her animals from their points of view and talked with her customers in laymen's terms they could clearly grasp. We also shared a few laughs together.

"There was the time, a bit later after Ava had moved back to Missouri, that a trucker had left off a hurt female bull terrier at her clinic up there. The dog was so dirty she was tan, and the guy did not know what kind of dog she was, just that he found her on the road. Ava instantly recognized her as a Bull Terrier, my favorite breed of dog. She named the dog 'Rosarita.' Because Rosarita reminded Ava about the place she liked most to be, Arizona, I agreed to take her. She shipped her off to me to care for her in a warmer environment. Her full name became 'Rosarita Chiquita Gonzales McCafferty!'

"Later, when visiting me, Ava had left some dirty clothes out on the floor, which she had readied for the washer. I, having learned Rosarita's habits, told her, 'Don't leave your unmentionables out and lying around like that.' You see, I already had found out the hard way that Rosarita had a taste for dirty panties, leaving me with a bunch of crotchless underthings … and I'm not even that kind of girl!

"Too late, Ava discovered that Rosarita had eaten the crotch out of her intimate items!

"We sure laughed hard about that. Still, to Ava, it was no big deal, but she did see the humor in it."

Also, that day, Arizona's infamous "dry heat" rescued them from the momentary setback. Ava donned a bathing suit that somehow had been spared the horrible ending of the other unmentionables and went outside to do some sunbathing. Minutes later, instead of scolding little Rosarita, she picked her up onto her lap and started singing *a cappella*, "Rosarita Rosarita, Rosarita Chi-qui-ta…" to the melody of Handel's *Halleluiah Chorus*!

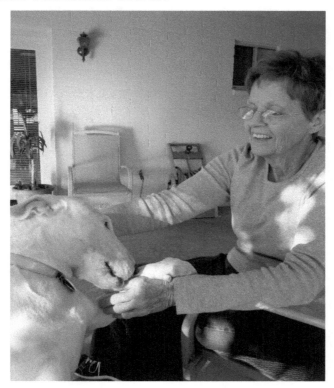

Nancy McCafferty & Rosarita Chiquita Gonzales McCafferty

Nancy and Ava's friendship outlasted the debacle of Rosarita's clothing antics. They would continue being friends through the time of Frick's pregnancy almost a decade later and through one of her visits for the Thanksgiving holiday, which had been coordinated around Ava's return to Arizona for an industry convention. And well beyond then.

Other events arrived on serious notes, like the rabbit that Nancy's cat "Earl" carried into her house the way a mama cat holds her young by the scruffs of their napes, a rabbit with a punctured neck. At first, Nancy thought, *Is that a RAT?* until Ava saw it and exclaimed, "OMG, it's a bunny!" Of course, they both wanted to do something to help the poor creature. Ava treated the bunny and left her with her friend, who inherited yet another animal to add to her menagerie.

Before that rabbit died from cancer a bit after Ava had treated her and left the area for Missouri again, Nancy had spent some time nurturing it as well as she had any of her other pets, and her friendships.

One time around 1991, the year the movie *Thelma & Louise* made hay at the box office, McCafferty and Frick shared a hilarious ride down Interstate 17 in an old, light-blue Chevy Impala sporting a white vinyl top and a fluffle of rabbits stretched across the bench seat in the back, during which McCafferty exclaimed, "Can you believe this picture of us with all these rabbits?!" They laughed for miles.

(Nancy and Ava are fast friends today. They spend Ava's birthdays together when their lives and work schedules allow for it.)

* * *

June 1986, was a pivotal moment in Ava's life and career. She had gone home to witness Lanie getting married and, while there, found that the family collectiveness and camaraderie left her wanting more of it. That, and a desire to get back into the horse world, gave her the impetus to talk to her Dad about her thoughts of moving back to Union from Phoenix. At the time, he was 59, and she 31.

She decided to return to Missouri and make it her home again, moved by her realization on her previous trip home that she still had three living grandparents and didn't want to

"... get 20 years down the road and say to myself, 'I wish I had spent more time with them.' Also, I had a-hankerin' to ride (horses) again."

> *"In his life, Dad never was one to deliberate a decision very long or to stifle what he saw as an opportunity. He swiftly went into his calculating mode: how could he help make this happen?*

> *"Two things had to have already shifted in our universe; one, that I had achieved my goal, so his prior doubts became moot; two, the willingness to confront where communication had been stifled on both our parts.*

> *"Dad met with Grandpa, and they agreed to assist me with a section of property they had along West Main Street."*

With that plan and a blueprint in hand, she initiated with her Dad the task of building her own practice to be called County Seat Animal Hospital & Services located in her home town of Union. Grandpa and Dennis oversaw construction of the building during the last vestiges of time that Dr. Frick had to work in Arizona.

> *"My ability to remain in Phoenix, gainfully employed, could not have happened without his love for this daughter and maybe, too, his missing me. Along with that were his dreams of future horse events, trail rides, and family outings to be shared.*

> *"The work became a labor of love and*
> *a win-win for everyone. Soon, I would be*
> *home, have my very own free-standing*
> *veterinary hospital with everything I*
> *dreamed of, and he and Mom would have*
> *more of their family together."*

For nine months, Dennis helped with local city and county permits, directed meetings with the contractor and sub-contractors, and ensured that what his daughter was describing she wanted and what they had in drawings were how things were coming along.

Then, in March of 1987, Ava packed up the Honda Prelude with one dog (Keoki), one cat (BeGee), and one rabbit (Finney) on board, opened the sunroof, and drove away, headed East. After two days of driving and overnight stops at friendly, one-pet-only motels—yes, she had two stow-aways, and each was litterbox trained, the clan hit the Missouri border at Joplin. Union was now a mere four hours away.

> *"My new adventure, a new way of life,*
> *was in the front windshield; what used to*
> *be… in the review mirror. Driving the rest*
> *of the way, I felt like, although I was going*
> *home, my heart was left in Arizona."*

The years to come would prove whether or not that was a real sensation.

* * *

CHAPTER 6: MISSOURI REDUX

Once Ava returned for good from her six-year stint in Arizona and was about to open the finished clinic in Missouri, she and Lanie started to enjoy each other's company as adults.

Lanie owned a four-year-old Appaloosa discovered to be, in her words, "a lazy horse." Ava, not having ridden any horse for a rather long stretch of time, asked Lanie to go with her on a ride, telling her that she wanted to ride the Appaloosa.

"Ava, I just told you she's lazy. I'm thinkin' of just sellin' her. You really want to ride her?"

"Well, sure, I do!"

Flabbergasted, Lanie handed over the reins and stood back, observing quietly as her older sibling mounted the slothful horse. Within minutes, Ava guided her chosen horse around effortlessly. Lanie had to admit to herself that somehow the two had connected; it sure seemed to her like they were communicating. She saw how the color-spattered Appaloosa took her rider's directions and no longer acted lazy. Remarkably, Lanie also observed that for the first time ever she had known her, Ava was utterly relaxed on top of a horse.

The filly's name, "Amiga" became a perfect fit in that magical moment. ("Girlfriend" in Spanish.) Without thinking about it, Lanie remembered that she had sensed agreement from the horse the first time she voiced the name to her. Apparently, Lanie possessed a bit of the same "touch" her sister had with animals.

Meanwhile, Ava took the Appaloosa's cooperation in stride:

"Amiga got me started at 32 [years].

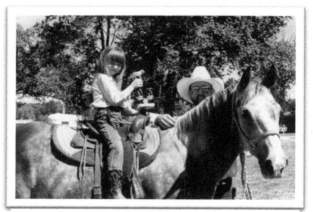

Lauren on Amiga, led by her Dad, Larry

She was calm, patient, and forgiving, taking whatever was the strongest cue I gave her, assuming that was what I meant and going with it. Maybe that only was a part of her easy-out nature, but it definitely worked for the two of us in our time. I out-grew her, eventually, and she became the caretaker of a young girl, Lauren Proemsey, once I advanced to my next horse, whom I called 'Poncey.'"

* * *

In the same year (1988), there came a time that Dr. Frick would not be able to ride a horse. Because of a painful incident away from the clinic, she would have to adjust her work schedule for a brief recovery time.

Participating in an adult women's soccer match on a local community playing field one evening, she maneuvering the black-and-white ball with her feet while hustling forward toward the net. From the outer corner of her right eye she spied an opposing player running straight at her, intent on more contact with her than the ball. She attempted to avoid the jarring contact that seemed inevitable. Too late, the other woman, a member of the dreaded Pacific (Missouri) team known for its roughneck style of play, body-checked her hard. Frick went down hard—not knocked-out cold but down for the count and unable to stand straight when she tried.

After the match ended, she returned home to try and rest through the night, hoping that a brighter morning would dawn to greet her. While the weather cooperated, her body wouldn't; she still could not stand up straight.

Frick canceled the day's appointments at her clinic and called the closest doctor's office she could think of in her state of mind.

Dr. Glen Calvin, not just an M.D. but also a Doctor of Osteopathy (D.O.), took on the emergency appointment with Frick. Once he had assessed her overall condition and the state of her injury, he adjusted her spine. (Understand, Dr. Frick had no prior knowledge of what a D.O. could do for another person, let alone for her distressed and painful body.)

Asked to, she immediately stood up straight! She was amazed. Here was something she hadn't known before.

"It was like Jesus had just saved me
with a miracle. I could stand up straight! It
was the best thing that ever had happened

*to me. Having an adjustment right after my
earlier horse-fall incident would have
helped me a lot, too."*

Dr. Calvin told her to go home and relax for the rest of the day, which she did do. The following day she was back at her clinic, working with her animal patients … and thinking about what possibilities the technology she had just experienced might have for her animal work. What had been her introduction to changing the locomotion of a human body, perhaps, could also benefit those of animals. Importantly, she also realized there was more to helping anyone in pain than a bottle or a pill prescription.

Of course, one adjustment was not enough for the severity of her condition. She returned several times to Dr. Calvin's office, although, oddly, he never charged her for the visits or therapy. This chain of events, possibly a sign that Providence watched over her professional career, motivated her to reach forward beyond the status quo of past training, her knowledge, and her work experience at her clinic. She continued to think and look outside of that box and into new areas of treatment for the animals under her care. These matters would be further enhanced by personal-life events yet to come and not far off from this moment in time.

Part of Ava's purpose for her return to Missouri was to get better and more comfortable about riding horses. Time spent working with them in her hours away from the clinic helped her to find a serene sense of peace, a feeling that she was more "one" with them as if she had done this before, a *déjà vu* sensation. She developed an uncanny sensitivity to their motions that combined with a prescient perception of their functions and posture. With that, she knew what they needed, what needed fixing.

Long trail rides afforded Ava ample time to reflect more on who and what a horse's spirituality might be, and what are his/her desires. Collating her equine thoughts and emotions, she wrote a beautiful treatise of her view of horses, faithfully presented here:

> *"There is something about a horse unique to itself. Little girls dream of them. For centuries, they have plowed our fields, pulled our wagons, carried couples to the altar, tended to kids, taken us away from danger, and gotten us back home. Horses have brought the bodies and souls of the rich and poor, and warriors, to battle.*

> *"The sound and rumble of the earth under the impact of thundering hooves leaves a heart speechless, stirring emotion to the inner core of both horsemen and horsewomen, including those unaware of the connection with their steeds.*

> *"Horses are empowering. They come with speed, grace, exhilaration, yet they are amusing, compassionate, and soulful. Horses speak with their eyes, and their eyes penetrate through our surfaces and reach into the unexplainable depths within us—places no other animal touches.*

> *"During the Great Depression, a simple racehorse, Sea Biscuit, took people a distance away from their strife, gave them purpose: something better to live for. To the struggling workers of America, at that time, he represented to the downtrodden and poor the hope that good*

things would happen after the bad. (They always do.)

"And who does not want to root for an underdog?

"Like most animals, the horse's connection to humans has been fraught with abuse. Yet, century after century, they, like ourselves and other animals, have returned to live among us time and again, forgiving the evils of the past for another chance to fulfill the wants, needs, and dreams of Man. It must be a part of their purpose for existing.

"For that opportunity to relive times gone by and to be reunited, moving together as Life, I am grateful. Still, all has not been a bed of roses, or peachy keen, when dealing with other spiritual creatures, because they have their mind about what they do or do not want to do, as well.

"Horses, for the most part, are large and strong. Their instincts are their inner truth, and they, unlike humans, always listen and obey. Horses, mules, and donkeys do not get in to quibbling about right and wrong the way we humans do. (Should I or should I not? What will others say?) With them, it is all about pure survival: how to avoid pain, escape a mountain lion jumping down from above on top of them, or that fight-or-flight mechanism that kicks in when a person

*gets on their back for the first time. With
horses, it's, '... get the hell out of there,
find a better place to be, and stick with the
herd.'*

"*That mindset challenges the horse
who is in constant discomfort and is
suddenly impinged upon by a saddle and
rider. Some do their best to ignore it and
go on. Some send gentle signals, at first
laying ears back, turning to frown as the
saddle is cinched, or swishing the tail
when asked to do a particular,
uncomfortable maneuver. Or crow
hopping: a style of bucking where a horse
arches its back and takes short, stiff hops,
hooves coming off the ground.*

"*When the rider fails to notice the
subtle hints and calm conversation, a
horse will resort to bucking. (And any
person who has ridden very much knows
where that can land us!)*

"*Compare that to a discussion
escalated to hollering. Even the most
caring and 'in-communication' equestrian
owner or trainer has, at times, fallen guilty
to this omission, and only awareness of the
early signs avoids the catastrophes.*"

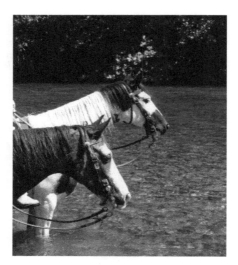

Horses on Jack's Fork River, Missouri

* * *

Ava was about to learn more than horse lore in the coming years of her lifetime. One English Lop rabbit had crossed with her the steppes and plains of New Mexico and Oklahoma from Arizona to Missouri. This male bunny had an unusual manner of making known his personal affinities and displeasures.

> *"Rabbits have their own unique personalities, as I learned when I became the veterinarian for a lop-rabbit breeder in Phoenix, Ross Malloy. This man had a soft heart. The first time we met, one of his champion Mini-Lop rabbits suffered a fractured rear leg and needed surgery. As luck would have it for me, I was the surgeon on duty that week. The orthopedic surgery involving the pinning of the leg went perfectly, and the rabbit went on to win more trophies.*

"Ross and I became friends. In 1986, he gave me my first English Lop kit rabbit, who had just been weaned. I named him 'Finney.'

"Finney quickly taught me his favorite reason for going out on my patio: he liked eating the eucalyptus leaves off the vine there, giving it a gentle pruning. Eventually, all the plants in the house, looking like Bonsai-trimmed hedges, were cleaned off as high up as he could stand on his rear legs.

"Finney would lounge on the sofa with me in the evenings as I watched TV or read a book. He had his spot next to my legs, occasionally hopping up to my chest to see what else was going on. After, he would leap off to the floor and race around the condo.

"How could I not love this guy?! Keoki (dog), BeGee (cat), and Finney all napped together; the latter two sharing a litter box in common without a fight. Life was so good the trio went with me on my move to Union in 1987.

"Later that summer, I began dating a guy. On a particular evening, by the time our date was over, it was late, and he ended up staying at my place for the night—something to which Finney was not accustomed.

"Someone is in MY place on MY bed next to MY Mom *must have been his thinking, because during the night this impeccably litter-box-trained rabbit littered the entire bedroom floor with pellets! No one could take a step for landing on one or more of the hard, dehydrated turds!*

"Finney had let me know his displeasure in no uncertain terms, and, to this day, I still laugh about him doing that."

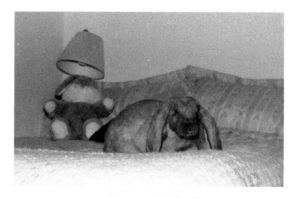

Finney on HIS bed!

* * *

Completing her first trip back to visit friends in Arizona in 1988 brought Ava a return home with 12 young English Lop rabbits in tow. Now her "family" had expanded drastically, marking the beginning of not only her Lops O' Fun Rabbitry company but also another learning curve involving a different species. For several years forward, she raised and showed the long-eared rabbits from Missouri to Ohio, Indiana, Michigan, Illinois, and Oklahoma. Her line of English Lops and her knowledge of how to help them medically elevated her to recognition from the leadership of the American Rabbit Breeder's Association (A.R.B.A.) before her interest factor ran its entire course.

One beautiful April Sunday several years later (1994) in Illinois, when she knew the rest of the Frick family were off riding horses at home in Missouri, Ava found herself sitting unhappily at a fairgrounds, waiting impatiently her turn to show. She took stock of her situation and decided it was time to "... *get out of the rabbit business and do more horsin' around.*"

The rabbit shows were a collection of the classes of rabbits; meat, fur, and fancy (the category in which the lops are placed). During one of those events in 1992, a trade of three rabbits and one breeding for a filly she would come to name "Twinkie," brought another winning smile to her face. And back to Missouri, she went!

> *"A woman was admiring my rabbits, and we started visiting. She told me of a six-month-old palomino filly that she was looking to sell. Before the day was done, we had a tentative agreement for me go home first and then drive back to Illinois and check her horse out..."*

By the time that took place more than a month had passed, because Ava wanted her dad to go with her and verify that this was a good idea and trade.

> *"... When we pulled up, the place had the appearance of difficult times: a fenced-in paddock with sheep, no grass that I can remember... and stuff here and there, which the sheep and this blonde, funny little horse climbed on..."*

She learned that this was where the young filly had been living all her life since weaned at two months.

> *"...It was not long before I knew I would be taking her home."*

At home, one sister said that "Twinkie" would be the right name for her, "Because she's yellow on the outside and full of crap in the middle!" And partially, that was true. Ava didn't entirely disagree with the assessment:

> *"She (the filly) had a good reason: she never learned horse etiquette... never had her mother nearby long enough to teach her right from wrong, or a herd to kick her around a little bit. Instead, she mimicked what she had learned. And all she had learned she knew from a flock of sheep, laying the ground for her unique and quirky personality..."*

Twinkie failed to understand how to get along with other horses through no fault of her own. Even though Ava took her in at only eight months of age, she already had developed certain behavioral traits that would never change.

> *"... But I loved her anyway, challenges aside."*

* * *

Twinkie

Dr. Frick's experiences with a variety of animals by this time—she had been in practice since 1980 and the '90s were upon her— taught her that each living creature brought lessons to her about virtues and qualities, which, in her previous thinking, almost exclusively had been assigned to human-to-human relationships, one being Patience.

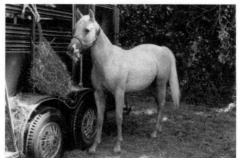

Twinkie

"Riding a horse can be an opportunity for people to learn patience; it was for me the day I tried to get one to cross a creek, and my mount was insistent that was not going to happen.

"I knew that getting frustrated would serve no purpose and that whipping with the reins was not the solution. I had learned the hard way the best approach was to train in a way that let the horse think he or she had decided to cross the creek or ditch. More often than not, that meant trotting, trotting, and more trotting close along the side of the obstacle. The more stubborn the horse, the longer the session. And at a trot, before long, sitting well in the saddle became a necessity; otherwise, bum, back, and legs ached for hours later."

One time, Frick rode with Dad and Lanie, and while their horses crossed the deep water-filled ditch, Twinkie with Ava aboard was having none of that.

> *"I told them to take off because we were going to have to reach an understanding. So, the trotting began and went on and on and on. Periodically, I stopped and looked across the abyss (as it appeared to Twinkie), while I talked to my mount. Logic, however, got me nowhere."*

The others, having traversed the whole trail, returned and stared at Ava and Twinkie from across the same water divide. To everyone's surprise, at that very moment, Twinkie changed her mind and suddenly leaped across the entire ditch, clearing the water by several feet!

Go figure.

By comparison, the two closest sisters' relationship was a lot smoother and more predictable than Twinkie and Ava. Lanie, like Ava with animals, self-motivated her pursuit of her artistic expressions: "Art was something I could always do. I took extra classes, and by high school, I was good at it. I just liked it."

Were these sisters two apples from different branches of the same tree? After all, they were making successful careers out of diverse passions, and Ava was among Lanie's best supporters and fans, buying six of her earliest wildlife portraits, which she painted on barn wood.

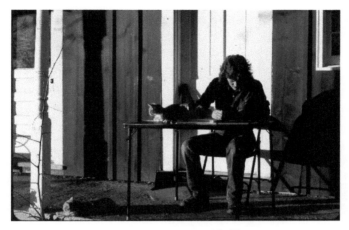

Lanie on art project, aided by two cats

For all the similarities, there were, at times, vast differences among the Frick family members, especially in matters of spirituality and religious belief. Ava's divergence began in her early years, arising (literally, at times) from her naturally intuitive perspectives about the living creatures around her and her out-of-body experience in the horse incident, besides the other mishaps, bumps, and bruises that anyone could attribute to growing up.

"Grandma Frick was Lutheran, and she went to church every Sunday. We were welcome to go along, but she never forced the idea. When Mom participated in religion, it was at the First Presbyterian Church, but she was not a regular.

"Neither Dad nor Grandpa had any attention in that direction, other than through their participation with the Masonic Lodge and 32nd Degree Scottish Rite. I don't recollect of Terry or Phyllis asking to go to church, but I did. I liked

*the warm feeling or caring for one another
that the church had.*

*"At Sunday school, we did arts and
crafts at young ages, so I got to create and
come home with a finished project to show
off. In later years, Sunday school led to
discussions that challenged my inner
spirituality. I had questions about self,
God, and who Jesus really was. I felt I was
looking for answers and help even at a
young age."*

* * *

The Frick family did not go to church every Sunday, and
sometimes months would pass without any of them in
attendance in the church pews. However, when Ava felt she
needed to be there, and she asked, Sarah always made it
happen.

Summer weeks in Bible schools for two faiths were fun
for Ava. She attended both Lutheran and Presbyterian,
feeling a personal connection to both. For her, church
attendance provided an inner something special that she
appreciated, and which was a result of the atmosphere,
music, smiles, people, pastors, and contents of readings from
the Bible.

*"I memorized the Lord's Prayer,
scriptures, and hymns in Bible school. Of
course, I especially enjoyed the ones that
included animals. In part, my Bible school
enjoyments were what led me to attend
Missouri Valley College, a Presbyterian-
affiliated college..."*

* * *

On the outside, Ava appeared content to live among her family and among her favored animals; inside, however, she searched for a higher meaning to her life and to living, perhaps, like many of us.

"Being active at the Trinity
Presbyterian Church throughout
veterinary college fulfilled my needs.
Moving with our diplomas to Arizona, as
we did after graduation, Bill and I did not
connect with a church, and maybe not
having religion in our daily lives played a
part in the struggle he and I had as a
married couple."

Once returned to Missouri, Frick quickly reconnected with the church she knew best. Fun, invigorating, and thought-provoking, the connection fueled a part of her soul that provided her extra guidance and purpose, as well as the opportunity to exhibit what meant most to her all along, the animals.

"Pastors changed, leaving some
interim ministers at the helm until
Reverend Charles and Malinda Spencer
landed there. They were my age and
igniting the church in a new way. Feeling
fulfilled, I took on being an Elder of the
church and a leader in Mission Moments
each Sunday. Also, I participated in
holidays, including decorating the annual
congregation Christmas tree.

"Everyone could bring an ornament
from home with which to decorate the
large sanctuary tree. When I came along,
my thought was that we should start doing

*themed decorations for a holiday. The
congregation went along with that, making
the trees be different and giving the pastor
a way to integrate a different message
each year.*

*"One year was an angel theme, and
all kinds of beautiful angels adorned the
tree. My angel? A pretty pink, winged pig
adorned with a halo!"*

* * *

The movie "*Babe*" is a good starting point to observe a variety of animal-communication styles if one looks past the animated lip and voice effects. Take note of eyes, tails, head positions, body postures, legs or wings, speed of motion … things like that. Additionally, note that animals can, at times, communicate verbally on another energy level termed variously 'soul-to-soul,' 'spirit-to-spirit,' 'prana-to-prana,' 'innate-to-innate, etc.'

Ralph was the first Vietnamese Miniature Potbellied Pig the Humane Society of Missouri took in at their Longmeadow Rescue Ranch just outside of Union. In Frick's words,

*"There was a lot not understood about
the term "miniature" back then. Such
animals, small at five months (25 pounds
or so) when compared to American hogs at
the same age (weighing in at 200-250
pounds), if continually fed and groomed
for years, can reach well over 300
pounds!"*

Who knew? Was Dr. Frick's first thought about Ralph. Because the Vietnamese slaughter and eat them young, she had no reason to believe any pig, especially this one, could get so large.

Ralph appeared on her horizon the day she was helping the Humane Society of Missouri Longmeadow Rescue Ranch with livestock care. Living on a farm as she did, made his adoption seem like the right thing to do. *Never mind the $750 adoption fee, he's the first of his kind, and, anyhow, he'll be little* she thought at the time.

Ralph turned out to be a fun and educational moment in time for Dr. Frick. As well, he added an entertainment factor for her clients and for locals in town. For example, a trio of bikers motoring through town stopped off at the White Rose Café on a day that table talk was all about Frick's "Ralph, the indoor pig." The three men then rumbled along west Main Street until they arrived at #1220—the clinic. Dressed in leathers and strolling into the place like they owned it, they asked to see the pig. Long story short, they had photos taken of themselves squatting beside Ralph right there in Dr. Frick's clinic!

Ralph soon exceeded 50 pounds, and his daily trips to the clinic ceased. Instead, Frick fixed up a hay mound in the barn where he hung out daily. At night, he made his way to the carport and went inside the house after Frick arrived from work.

Now, imagine this in a kitchen: two dogs, one cat, one large, potbellied pig with a kitten perched atop his back all lined up for supper. And Ava cooking dinner for the whole lot! (The rabbit, of course, off somewhere else!)

After each evening meal, like clockwork, Ralph retired for the night to his personal *indoor* bed in Ava's bedroom. In the morning, out he went.

Ralph was particular about his beds, too. Every now and

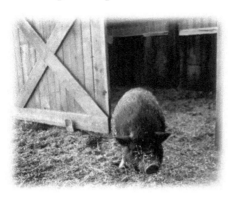

Ralph

again, after Ava cleaned up the barn and refreshed his hay mound… *"Oh, the trauma of it all!"*… in protest, Ralph moved away and circled the enlarged ranch-style house, grumbling and complaining like only a heavyweight alien pig could. Obviously distraught about the changes and rearrangements being made to "his" furnishings and sleeping quarters, he turned three full roundabouts by the time she finished her chore and had his new "sheets" in place. That's when Ralph would make his way back to the barn, sniff and inspect her handiwork, and inevitably lay himself down again for a long-awaited nap. On cold and freezing days, he would hide in it, invisible to the world. When Ava walked into the barn and called his name to see if he was there, she heard a grunt and saw the hay mound bounce. Ralph was a far cry from the tiny, winged "Angel" pig that adorned the church's Christmas tree!

> *"That pig was not too far out of the box for me, because in the spring came the Blessing of the Animals event to which I was permitted – actually requested – to bring some of my animals for the children's sermons. Included in my usual list were an English Lop rabbit, a dog or two, and one of my pot-bellied pigs! (Yes, even Ralph or Agnes strolled down the aisle following the popcorn trail!)"*

Frick's menagerie guaranteed a jam-packed sanctuary each season as the parishioners filed in anxious to see who would be on display and what the kids would say and do in response to the minister's message to them.

"Following the 'Angel' year, our theme was the 'Creche' - [a depiction of] baby Jesus in the manger. When Reverend Spencer made that announcement, he stuck in an addendum, 'And, Ava, no baby animals portrayed as Jesus, please.'

"The whole church burst into laughter, for everyone, including me, knew that could happen! Yet, that was my first year to not have any animal on the tree."

* * *

By 1990, Dr. Frick's County Seat Animal Hospital had a deserved reputation for the good among the local area's residents. Hers was the first in the county to have an in-clinic laboratory blood testing system that yielded blood results within an hour or two. She was in demand and working many hours around the clock well before present-day technological advances and devices. Telephones were ubiquitous; a phone at work, another at home, and payphones strategically located around local towns—the latter only convenient to the doctor if she was already in the city and happened to have a full cupful of quarters, dimes, and nickels in her truck. A pager connected to a system controlled by the Radio-Comm Company in nearby Krakow allowed her to take calls day and night. After hours, the clinic phone forwarded to their service. They answered for the doctor, jotted down important information, and dispatched a phone number that showed up on Frick's pager window for her to handle. A difficult or complicated incoming call required her talking to the answering service first.

"A particular nighttime emergency call sticks in my mind, one that forever changed how I approached my examinations, especially during a stressful situation.

"A dog had been hit by a car. Carried in recumbent, I took all the traditional assessment steps, making a determination that he would live, except that he needed some emergency care, and the fractured leg would need surgery.

"An estimate was worked up. The owners agreed to save their friend, and a deposit was made. The dog was stabilized for that day and had a surgery planned for the next morning. Because of his condition upon arrival, we kept him quiet and lying down.

"In wanting to not stress him further, I had failed to thoroughly examine every leg. The next morning after his sedation and while prepping for surgery, I found that I had made a terrible error. Not only did he have a fractured left rear leg but also a broken humerus in the right foreleg!

"Of necessity, there were two parts to my enacted solution. First, I accepted my mistake and took responsibility for it, and repaired the front leg at no cost.

"This was his lucky day: he would live to run and play. Had the owners known about it in advance, they would not have

been able to afford everything, and the dog would have been euthanized.

"Part Two was to change the operational basis that got me into that predicament. Thereafter and forever, my mantra was to look at the obvious last, for it was the not-so-obvious that could be missed!

"I still practice that way today with my physiotherapy patients. It works!"

* * *

Not every rotation in Dr. Frick's day-to-day business affairs and job positions was a bed of roses or an enthusiastic charge of the light brigade against the common enemies of animal illness and disease. Mere living brings wins and losses to everyone, and she, too, could not escape every obstacle presented on her journey. Regardless, she still had to perform at her top-shelf level of ability and acumen every hour of every day. That said, many days brought her unforgettable rewards for a job well done.

"An old farmer brought his favorite friend in to see me, a Beagle-mix. She had been sick for a few weeks and was growing weak. Fortunately, my clinic's laboratory system could run blood tests and get results the same day. As I explained what I was thinking and wanted to do, the farmer constantly stroked her body.

"Suddenly, tears started rolling down his cheeks. He began apologizing that 'she is just a dog' and he didn't know why he was crying.

*"You see, back when he was young,
many people on farms grew up with the
mindset that the house was for humans,
and all animals were kept outside. He
seemed one from that generation. To him,
spending money on a dog was foreign.*

*"Still, he was thinking with his heart,
which would not let him leave her be sick.
She had loved him unconditionally, and
that love had melted through. In return, he
loved her.*

*"I assured him that it was good to
have a friend that he enjoyed that much
and wanted to help.*

*"She ended up staying with us for a
few days. When she left with her 'Dad,'
there she was, sitting right next to him in
the front seat of his pick-up truck. And
down the road, they went... maybe with a
piece of my heart, too."*

Before the new decade arrived, another significant event
would come to pass: the fulfillment of a promise Dr. Frick
had made to her local-area neighbors and friends. For several
years prior to 1987, her sister Phyllis and her husband, along
with a group of others with similar concerns for the animals
in the local area, sensed a need for a way to protect and
rehabilitate the stray animals that populated the region.
Eventually, they ceased their procrastination and established
a 501(c)(3) for what they called the Franklin County
Humane Society (FCHS) and commenced a series of
fundraising events to help pay for the assistance given to lost
and unwanted pets. The group formally opened a bank

account with the United Bank of Union, and their hard-raised funds were deposited there.

Coincidentally, Dr. Frick had decided in June of 1986 to end her extended stay in Arizona and return to Missouri. By March 1987, she hung out her shingle as a working, local veterinarian. As part of her Grand Opening, local radio, news media, and newspapers welcomed her, calling her the "other" Vet Doctor—there had been only one in the area for about 30 years! Headlines read "Hometown Girl Comes Home," but everyone on the telephone gossip line—what community didn't have one of those back then?—wondered what the "new" Veterinarian would offer beyond the other doctor's menu.

Besides new technology equipment, Dr. Frick brought her ability to perform a variety of surgeries and, among other skills, her unique manner of communicating with her patients (the animals). In time, one major St. Louis media source dubbed her, "St. Louis' 'Animal Whisperer.'"

Speaking to the press in an interview, Dr. Frick went out on a limb, telling a reporter, "One of my goals is to establish a Franklin County Humane Society office here."

(After all, she had worked at one in Arizona and had the experience to know what they needed and how to run one.)

Time pushed on. Days and months slipped by without much progress toward that goal until one day in November that one of Dr. Frick's customers inquired about her pledge.

Dr. Frick realized instantly that she had no choice: *"I have to do this now."*

Fundraising through events, newspaper articles, radio announcements, and media-appearance interviews continued once Frick was on the Board of Directors alongside John Stoltz, DVM, and other caring individuals and business owners of the community. But an actual location would not be found for the service until 1993, once again involving Dr. Frick in the solution to the problem.

It wasn't like Ava didn't have enough on her hands with the clinic, staff, raising and showing rabbits, her horse and pets; and being president of the Franklin County Humane Society, besides spending time with her grandparents. She did get it in her mind that the community needed an indoor training, boarding, and grooming facility. Before anyone knew it, in 1989, she began work on another project of creating, designing, theming, and building something new that she called "Pet Station."

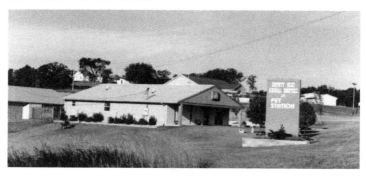

County Seat Animal Hospital with new Pet Station behind it

The new facility would include a drive-up, drop-off, pick-up window for those nasty weather days and nights that can beset Missouri in late-fall and winter months! It opened in 1990. Building a second business when her clinic was just barely off the ground by three years, one could say, was par for the Dr. Frick course: the 'ready – fire – aim" part of her never waited for much. She would find, however, that this time, she bit off more than she really wanted to chew. This new project added a lot of stress, despite that she was the one creating it. After three years of investing her blood, sweat, and tears into establishing this new type of pet care in Union, it was time for her to sign off on the idea.

However, all was not lost. This facility provided the perfect venue for the soon-to-be FCHS shelter after she offered to sell at face value the building that housed Pet Station. Another dream was now completed. There would be a building to support better care, a place for unwanted, abused, and lost pets in Franklin County to enter—one better than any of the city pounds ever were able to provide.

Despite her knowing that any competing doctor could put in a bid for the FCHS animal-care contract, Frick listened to the outcry which declared the objection that her clinic's on-site location gave her an unfair advantage to pick up clients from the FCHS. She promptly resigned her position on the FCHS Board and passed the gavel to the next generation.

(In 2004, FCHS officials, recognizing the role she had played in putting the organization on the map, awarded Dr. Ava Frick the Visionary Award for her volunteer work and assistance. And in October 2008, she received the Emeritus Director Award for outstanding dedication to the Franklin County Humane Society.)

* * *

CHAPTER 7: COWGIRL UP!

The next decade began with Dr. Frick finding a new companion, which suited her just fine.

"When I came home from work one day, a seven-month-old Spitz Pekinese-mix dog came trotting out of the carport, saying, "Hi, I live here!" I looked at him and said, "That's funny, I live here too." He had a collar and a St. Charles County rabies tag—a long way from Union.

"No one ever came looking, and he never left, so, he became mine. I named him, 'Joey.'

"Joey was the best dog ever, not that Keoki wasn't a good dog. Or 'Cheerio,' also a Corgi, but different. He got excited whenever I had a late-night emergency. He sat by me as I took the phone call, following up the two a.m. pager. With my hanging up, he always knew if I was going back to bed or going to get dressed. Maybe I had used the same words every time, and he learned them? *thought I.*

"If I was going, that meant he was going for a truck ride. Just as I placed the

phone in its cradle, he would start dancin'
his happy dance! If not, he'd quietly amble
back to his bed.

"At the clinic, Joey acted the
ambassador, welcoming owners, and then
quietly walked into the exam room and
found his usual space under the counter.
His presence alone calmed first-time
visitors. The 'regulars' all looked forward
to their furry friend being there, assuring
them with his calmness that all would be
fine. On days when a bossy dog thought it
could get in Joey's face and start
something, he would just turn his head
away, diffusing the advance.

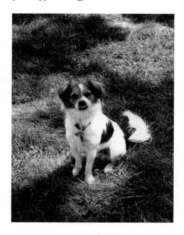

Joey

"Joey not only had etiquette but also
know-how: he was the star of trick-dog
classes!

"Joey had appeared out of nowhere at
seven months, and one wintry night of his

*17th year, he simply disappeared while we
were down at the folks' place in Licking,
far from anywhere. I knew he was deaf and
couldn't see in the dark. I had asked
everyone to tell me if they saw him by the
door wanting out because I needed to go
with him. He joined us for supper, but, by
bedtime, was nowhere to be found.*

*"We called and called. We got out the
'Gator' [six-wheel farm vehicle] and went
around the fields and through the woods,
but all we brought in was the cows. The
next morning, Lanie and I went out early
looking for him on horses. I pictured him
curled up next to a tree. No Joey. He was
gone without a trace.*

*"Even this day as I write about him, I
get choked up fighting back the tears. How
could he care for me so much that he
would choose to make a quiet exit?"*

* * *

Even though this event was yet another loss with no
good-bye possible, Dr. Frick was by now better equipped to
deal with it. She knew that Joey was a spiritual being and
that he had his own choices to make. Never a problem in life,
he had not wanted to be one at the end of his trail.

*"Funny, though, I don't remember the
day, date, or exact year that Joey left me. I
know that night was cold and ... (oddly)
thinking of it ... [I] can't remember the
date Dalton and I said good-bye to our
beloved 14-year-old cat, Oliver. He was
eight when I brought Dalton home from*

the hospital—unusual for an adult cat to decide his job was to be with the baby, maybe because Dalton rarely cried. But, no matter wherever Dalton was, Oliver would place himself right next to him. After doing surgery twice on Oliver's mouth for cancer, it returned once again. Dalton, only six years old, saw this time that Oliver was having more difficulty eating and being comfortable and asked me, "Please, Mama, don't do any more surgery."

"I do recall that it was sunny the day at 15 ½ years that I walked with Cheerio to the vet and bid our years together adieu, but not the day or date. And the day Token, a magnificent black-tabby, was killed on the road I thought he never crossed? ... I know it not.

"Maybe this was a way for me to be able to get past those days and dates, without reliving my grief; otherwise, I would be in a constant sad state, given all the animals and loved ones I have lost over the years. Still, when I think of them, it's about their lives, not their deaths.

"Memorials should be on the birthday, not the death day. It's more about the coming and being. Separation is painful and, while death is a marker to an era, it's a departure with the uncertainty of when we might meet again. Legacies begin with birth, grow and thrive on a primary purpose and how determined we are to fulfill it at the requests of everyone's God

to be kind, to share and care about
everything and everyone around us."

*   *   *

Frick was about to see significant changes that would alter the course of her personal life in ways she could not imagine. Those changes would revise her entire approach to her career.

"Lanie and I decided one day to take
some excess tack to the sale-barn
auction—horse and tack night followed
small-livestock night.

"We found resting in the back stalls a
small tan goat with a huge oval, numbered
sticker plastered across his forehead—the
only place a goat could not rip it off. The
label was so large that he had to raise his
head and peer out from under it like he
was wearing a broad-brimmed visor in
order to see us. He was so cute. I inquired
at the office about him because, by now, I
had decided that he needed a good home
rather than be sold and end up who knows
where. Most likely, his new home was
going to be mine. As it turned out, other
folks also had asked about him. The
previous night's purchaser had left him
behind 24 hours earlier; the auctioneers
were going to put him back on the sales
block.

"After the horses and the tack were
sold, the time had come to bid on the baby
goat. Three of us were upping the bid: me,
another family, and the "Killer" (what we

called the man who takes animals to slaughter). We continued to raise the bid until the Killer dropped out. When he did, I decided the little goat was safe. The price hit $45, and I went out.

"As I left the auction barn, I walked over to the family who won the bidding war and gave them my business card, telling them, 'He is still intact. Billy goats get rather stinky and ornery, so you may want to get him castrated. I would be happy to help you with that.'

"Long story short, a few months later, the same goat was on the clinic's books for his 'coming-out party'—how I kindly refer to neutering or castration services. (Note: Many men, I have noticed, have a difficult time comfortably handing their dog or cat over for that event. Saying the words 'coming-out party' makes it much more tolerable for them, and they often leave chuckling.)

"Like a dog, 'Bart' walked well on a collar and leash as if he had been doing that his whole life. He was a little guy who carried a big scrotum, but his lifestyle was about to change!

"After the procedure, we never heard from his owners until Spring of the following year when a phone call came in from them. They were moving to Arizona, and they asked me if I would be able to

take care of him until they got settled in there.

"'Sure!' I told them, thinking, after all, I live on a farm, and he's such a cute little guy.

"The day the family came to leave him with me, they arrived in a four-door sedan packed with four people and one enormous goat. The little guy was not so little anymore.

"Standing about hip high at his back (my hips and I am long-legged) with his Nubian ears drooping, his glances dart left to right. I try to take a quick assessment and figure out what is going on with him, but I am shell-shocked: no way had I ever expected that he was going to be this large!

"I take the lead rope and show his family around the place. They promise that as soon as they get settled, they will be back to get him. We say our good-byes, and I take Bart to the barn.

"Easter comes, and they send Bart a card with a message of how they miss him. Next, Halloween arrives, and again Bart receives mail from them: 'BOO!' Two months later, a Christmas card labeled Season's Greetings from Phoenix arrives, but that was the last he ever heard from his 'family.'

"Shortly after, Bart becomes an official, permanent resident of 'Ava's Clan.'

"If nothing else, Bart was a typical goat, an entertainer. Yet, in my presence, he copped an attitude with some regularity, likely easily attributable to the day he lost his jewels at the hands of a surgeon: ME!

"Bart could be very serious about his displeasure at the memory, too, rearing up with his head cocked sideways and lunging forward and coming down hard right in front of me, but only because I had stepped back quickly enough. He would preferably have made contact, of that I'm sure!

"Throughout his life, Bart tended to like men better. And about this time (1991), Tony Kuenzel came into my life from the rodeo and country-western dance-floor circuit."

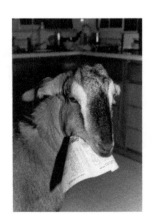 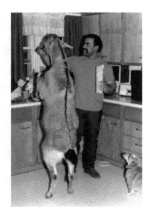

Kuenzel had been a champion wrestler in his school days and had moved on to a less-forgiving sport in his adult years, finding happiness in eight-second increments atop cantankerous, loud, ornery bulls on display in local rodeo rings ... until a dropped-ear goat came along and took a liking to him.

> *"Tony and Bart got along well. One year the Franklin County Humane Society was having a Dog-Walk fundraiser, so we decided that Bart was due for an outing. On the way over, he rode in the front of the truck at shotgun. Once there, walking him was a lot easier than the struggles many of other folks experienced with their dogs tugging and pulling their owners left and right. Twice we heard people say, 'What kind of a dog is that?' (Too funny: because it was a dog walk, they believed every animal must be a dog. LOL)*

> *"Deer season on the outskirts of town with a sizeable tan-colored goat who could be mistaken for a deer meant that Bart got fitted for a bright orange vest. He wore it, too, albeit with some disdain, but that didn't stop him from walking down the gravel driveway and across Springfield Avenue to Platt's Nursery, a hunters' check-in point. There, Bart, either attracted by all the abnormal hustle and action or, perhaps, the sight of what might be kin, decided to assess the situation more closely for himself by himself.*

> *"Shortly thereafter, a page from my answering service tells me to return a call*

to the number listed on the screen. Soon enough, I discover it's Gene Platt's number. Bart had walked in the front door of the nursery and was running an inspection in the place ... Bart style: goats and greenery intended for sale and profit do not go well together. Goats love to eat all kinds of weedy, stemmy plants. A forté is poison ivy, though they are not much for grass.

"In the nursery, whenever someone tried to get Bart under control, he reared up and showed his 'No, you don't!' side. I

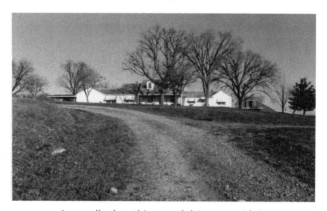

Ava walked up this gravel driveway with Bart in tow

grabbed the leash, walked down the driveway, and fetched him home – a daring feat that was the talk of their shop for some time to come!"

* * *

The only thing constant in Frick's life at this point was change. Wal-Mart came in and pitched a bid for buying up the Frick farm on the west side of Union. Since she was the caretaker there, living in the old farmhouse after Grandma and Grandpa moved into assisted-living facilities, the proposition forced her to hunt for a new place to live. When Wal-Mart changed their minds and located their new store on another property on the east side of town, Frick by then already had another home out on Camp Mo-Val Road, to which her animals moved, including three horses, two pigs, two dogs, two cats, and, of course, Bart.

"Camp Mo-Val was further out of town and contained an earth-shelter house, a pond, and a tall, three-sided metal building, which Tony and I turned into a barn. With the variety of animals, Lotta Bars Ranch became the name of our new establishment. We added an arena or two and fencing for pasture, and we were set. Or so we thought.

"One night, I got home late from work. It was pitch black outside. When I walked into the house and flipped on the light, I saw the place had been ransacked! Suddenly, out of the bedroom ran Bart, looking for an exit. The dang goat had figured out how to work the door handles and had gotten into the house, but the wind had closed the door behind him.

"Bart had gotten into the cabinet where the cereal and raisins were stored, had helped himself to three varieties, and finished off the grapes. He also had nibbled the tops of the dried-flower arrangements I had in the house, leaving only stems. Eyeing the sheets, I realized

*that he had settled himself in the middle of
the bed for a nap!*

*"After a couple more incidents of him
coming in to visit while we lived there, we
decided it was time to install an Invisible
Fence, which we did differently than most
people would. Most people put an electric
fence around the perimeter of their
property to keep their dogs in. We had to
put it around the house and patio deck to
keep the goat out. From then on, Bart wore
the collar, standing just out of range,
twisting his head, shaking his body, and
looking at us in disgust. For us, though,
life was a lot safer that way since the only
place he could get me cornered was when I
was in a horse stall at the barn."*

* * *

Doing a strictly dog-and-cat veterinary practice, at
times, could become mundane, but Dr. Frick solved that
situation by moving in different circles of activity.

*" 'Variety is the spice of life!' as the
saying goes. Adding rabbits and other
pocket pets, like the injured chinchilla at
the FCHS, which we nursed back to
health; the discarded guinea pig I named
"Skittles;" Reba the rat, a few birds here
and there (one, we radiographed and
splinted a broken leg).*

*"Zebra Finches decorated the clinic
colorfully, and pot-bellied pigs brought
us a variety of new and educational*

experiences ... though none quite as
unique as the herd of llamas!

"To Everything, There Is a
Season..." sang *The Byrds in '65. The*
high-season for llama popularity was the
'90s. That's when a herd owner living
near Augusta across the Missouri river,
found me. Before that, the only exposure
I ever had to this Camelid species was
the young male, Spitz, at Pet-A-Pet.

"We had to be fast enough to catch
him though, because of his distinct sound,
the look in his eye whenever he zeroed in
on someone to mount, and his boot-
scootin' across the shavings-covered
cement! Needless to say, his compatibility
with the public became a liability, and he
was relocated to a lifestyle farm better
suited to his proclivities!"

* * *

The Augusta llama farm set on rolling hills amid tall
trees and minor fencing—llamas respect a rope, unlike
bison, for example. The '30s cow barns had some wear and
tear, but they were adequate for the llamas. And two, trusty
Great Pyrenees protected the herd from villainous coyotes,
wolves, and the occasional pack of wild dogs.

God provides species with unique qualities for optimal
survival. A prey bird's vision enables it to see a ground
rodent from several miles up in the sky. A dog's snifter
smells 10,000 times beyond a human's.

And then there are llamas.

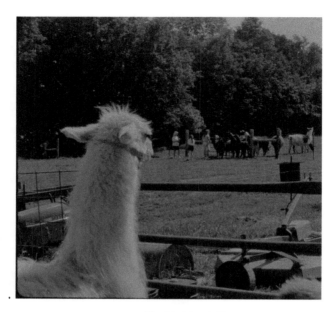

The Matriarch Llama

Llamas' large, beautiful eyes on the sides of their heads have a visual range of almost 360 degrees—a slight shift of the head peruses the rest and detects danger. A llama herd has a leader, usually the senior female, a matriarchal "queen" of sorts. Such was the case of the one Dr. Frick met: tall, statuesque, she carried herself with an air of royalty accented by her pure white color (reminiscent of sashaying Victorian Queens in England).

One early-summer *Saturday* morning—hey, that's how country veterinarians do it—Dr. Frick's mission was to draw some blood on the young ones, do some standard parasite treatments and vaccinations, and scoot. Time would be tight; Tony and she were headed to a Bar-be-que that afternoon. The doctor would have to get home on time, switch vehicles, and then be on their way.

> *"Upon my arrival, the herd owner*
> *already had sorted them, a good and bad*

thing; good for me, less waiting; bad because this was NOT a regular routine, the llamas were on edge.

"S.O.P. (Standard Operating Procedure) when working with llamas is never, I repeat, NEVER look one in the eye. The result can be getting spat upon.

"As we set up to get workin' on the "cria" (American Spanish for "baby llama"), they sent out distress calls. The matriarch began pacing back and forth on the other side of the isolated working pen inside the barn. I was diligent and time-efficient with each cria to minimize everyone's stress, and the farm owner was doing her best to keep the group calm, especially the leader, now focused on the stranger-danger present in her midst.

"About to switch out to cria number three, I stood up and turning toward my left, a small corner of my right eye scanned the outer perimeter and caught her eye. That wasn't meant to happen!

Too late! That female was locked, cocked, loaded, and ready to fire. And fire she did! There was no ducking. Frick was hit. Not even Wyatt Earp could stave off this indefensible attack.

"This was not a simple spit; this was regurgitation—a heave of her entire green, acidic, fetid stomach contents in one lump sum! She had unloaded all over

*the front of me ... my hair, eyelids, shirt
... annihilated!*

*"And STIIINNKK?! You can't
imagine unless you've experienced it
first-hand.*

*"The stench permeated the barn, the
owner, and me. All the other llamas
instantly knew what had happened: She
had retaliated ... from only five feet away
like a water hose turned on full blast!
OUCH!*

* * *

The only thing left was the crying, and Frick had no time for that. Wiping off the worst, she got on with finishing the task at hand, drove 45 minutes home with the windows down, wearing dirty, stinky clothes. At home, she showered, but the smell lingered. The shirt never came clean of the green stain.

Tony laughed, as Ava pondered her lesson, concluding aloud, *"Never plan a bar-b-que and llamas on the same day.* 'To everything, there is a season… a time to laugh, a time to weep.' *I did some of both that day."*

* * *

Memories dot anyone's life with horses, including Ava's fun times with friends, events of skillful accomplishments by riders and horses working as teams— dressage, hunter-jumper, ranch riding, reining, or cutting; other times, beating a time clock or winning a race by two lengths. The similarity to them all is time spent in the saddle compared to on the ground. But, unless a rodeo saddle-bronc or bareback rider, they really don't expect to end up on the ground, though eventually, that happens to everyone. Some more than others.

Ava's fourth-grade event was the first, not the last, of her "horse incidents." Many were half-falls whereby leaning too far to one side made abrupt landings less harmful. (Her sister Terry once held on long enough to find a soft landing spot—kerplunk!—her pride getting hurt more than her heinie.)

> *"Back when I was living at the old homestead, before Tony and I started dating, I joined Dad, Lanie, and a couple of other friends, Gail and Helen, on a weekend ride to Shawnee National Forest in southern Illinois. After breakfast, we saddled up, bent on a leisurely trail ride..."*

The caravan consisted of three trailers with living quarters, custom-made for tooling across Missouri to southwest Illinois. Ava rode her 15.3-hand Bay Appendix, a Quarter Horse/Thoroughbred cross, "Poncey" (her steed after selling Amiga). Spring to early summer temperatures had set in late enough in the year to not need coats and early enough to not pack a lot of water in the saddlebags. The horse flies weren't bad, and the itch weed wasn't out yet. Dressed in shirts, jeans (overalls for Dennis), boots, and cowboy hats, they were suitably decked out.

> *"... Picking up a few other riders we had met at camp the night before gave us a group of eight. We had made our way three hours out, had stopped for lunch, and were on our return to camp, going single file on a dirt path through an open field. Dad was the scout in the lead with one or*

*two of the other riders. I was in the fourth
position, and one of the new cowgirls filled
in behind me, followed by Lanie and Gail.*

*"I was having a conversation with the
person behind me, when all of a sudden, I
jolted and was propelled out of the saddle.
That much I remember, the rest is a blank.*

*"As the story goes, I'm told there was a
reasonably large stick in the path, which
the three horses and riders in front of me
had ignored. My mare stepped on one
end of the stick, and the other end shot up
and jabbed her in the belly, startling her
all to heck. A lunge, a buck, and she was
rider-free. A couple more kicks and
running circles, and she stopped.*

*"Everyone, by then, had dismounted.
Lanie sent Dad to fetch the horse, and
Gail—she had been a Korean military
mash surgical nurse and had seen many
war wounds—went in to combat mode…"*

Gail was quite something! She wore her hair in short-
cropped military-style right into her mid-50s and was about
10 years older than Ava; short and Gestapo-ish; a kind of no-
kidding-around woman—you know, confident and capable.
Gail could be funny when she lit into someone with her
gravelly smokers' voice and laugh.

*"There I lay totally knocked out,
unconscious about what had transpired.
The next thing I remember is looking at
Gail, inches away from my face, staring
down at me, waiting to see what my*

pupils were going to be like the instant
my eyes opened. My first words were,
'What are you doing there?' to which she
laughed heartily, explaining what I was
doing on the ground with her face in
mine: 'I'm waiting to see if you're okay.'

"Once I got my faculties re-oriented, the
others helped me up. Blood covered my
face and neck. Of all places to land, my
head had managed to find the only rocks
in the field!

"Not too far away, a creek flowed, so
Gail and Lanie helped me to the water.
After some appropriate splashing, Gail
determined that all of the blood had come
from the back of my head.

"I felt okay to ride, but we were an hour
and a half from camp and another hour
and a half from any town. Cowgirl-up!
was what I had to do."

Back at camp, Gail and Ava walked to the rustic
bathroom for a closer look. The wound was a sizeable three-
corner tear all the way to the skull, not that there is much
mass on the head between skull and scalp. With a mirror and
Gail pulling her blood-pasted hair aside, the duo could see
Ava's skull seams.

"Now I am feeling a wee bit queasy.
Where initially I was fine for Gail to
close the wound by tying my long hair in
a knot, now I am reconsidering that
something should be done about it.

*"We load up and head to the nearest
town, looking for a veterinary clinic
where I can beg off some lidocaine,
sutures, betadine scrub, sponges, needle
holders, and forceps and let Gail relive
her earlier days as a Medic. I wholly
trust her. Unfortunately, it was a
Saturday, and by the time we arrived, the
clinic had closed.*

Remember, this was before cell phones. They had no
way to pre-call anyone anywhere in "the good old days!"

*"We drove on, eventually finding a
doctor's office right before their closing.
Though the doctor was gone, a nurse
practitioner was still there, and he was
up for performing the surgery. With each
of his passes through my scalp, I sensed
the trembling of his hands. Maybe he was
aware that as a veterinarian, I had
definitely done more surgeries than he,
or maybe Gail's presence and eyes
emitted an air of her seniority over a
surgery table."*

Right then, Ava wished she held the needle holders and
forceps in her hands. Stitched up, and frustrated about the
lack of surgical finesse shown by the nurse practitioner, she
was once again in the truck on their way back to join the
others. An hour and a half later, the group made it back to
camp in time for supper with a new story to tell at the
campfire. From then on, Ava never left home horseback-
bound without her own emergency kit replete with
everything needed to do laceration repairs.

* * *

In 1994, Tony and Ava tried to start a family but lost a baby to a miscarriage. By year's end, the family's outlook looked bleak. Still, past the unpalatable turn of events, the music and musicians they always fell back on—Garth Brooks, Clint Black, Travis Tritt, Marty Stuart, Dwight Yoakam, Alan Jackson, Aaron Tippin, Suzy Bogguss, Holly Dunn, K.T. Oslin, and Lee Ann Womack, to name a few, all decidedly country/western stars, became emotional outlets for whenever the couple tried to make something better of their life together on a dance floor or outside on horseback.

Right then, a light of hope entered her life. Dr. Frick was about to meet someone capable of shouldering the load of some of the burdens of the business; someone who could tune in to Frick's spiritual leanings and wavelengths she shared with animals, Mary Lenau.

Mary Lenau owned a veritable menagerie of animals at home, including four dogs, two horses, and 15 goats—meat goats suitable for breeding. Now recently moved from St. Louis proper to rural Union after discovering and purchasing the farm she wanted, the next goal on her agenda was locating a new and nearby job position. She was no longer willing to endure the time-consuming daily commute to and from the city of St. Louis, and no longer willing to spend any more time working in clinics that still operated "old-school," that were "inside the box," so to speak.

Dr. Frick's ad for a veterinarian technician (Vet-Tech) ran at the same time that Lenau started searching the help-wanted columns. Lenau applied for the position and right away got the green light from her new boss, because she and Frick immediately discovered understandings between them on more than one level: they both owned horses; both had cats, dogs, and goats; both were similar in age at 40-something—only a year apart. Finally, each still yearned for that elusive "something more out of life" that so many of us crave at different times of our lives.

Straight away, Frick noticed that Lenau was capable of managing the technical side of her business. Putting her in charge there allowed the doctor to rotate with her new assistant, freeing her own time while boosting Lenau's confidence in the bargain.

According to Lenau, "Ava was experiencing high turnover rates from employees because she was strict and stuck to demanding of her staff high moral and ethical standards, as well as competent technical capabilities. Her staff relations were not about being personable, but about what helped the animals most. Lots of employees would get intimidated at first."

The metaphor "If you can make it in Manhattan, you can make it anywhere"—in this case, Union—applied to Frick's clinic personnel, but only for those who lasted long enough to experience stellar outcomes from Dr. Frick's setting the standards bar high.

It didn't hurt that Lenau, too, was of German descent, enabling her and Frick to get along well despite occasional rough patches.

"We worked out a system that smoothed the office waters: a note written in large letters pushed a new clinic policy that counted for the whole staff, including the doctor, 'Yell on paper but *talk* to me,'" Lenau recalled.

Soon, staffers and the doctor added other routine group activities in the form of trail-rides and company parties, replacing what had been a nagging problem: how to find the right balance between work and socializing. Up to that point, a maze of dead-end directions, unpredictable reactions, and uncomfortable maneuverings had brought, at times, morasses of sudden emotional outbursts that challenged everyone. Too much seriousness had invaded and dropped a blanket over purpose, driving office stats in the wrong direction. Something had to change.

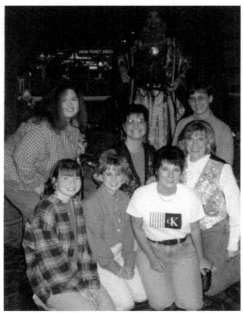

Staff with Dr. Ava in Las Vegas

Fortunately, holiday parties and impromptu weekend overnight trips that included floats on rafts down lazy rivers melded the personnel into a team that knew when to have fun and when to wax serious and perform the needed work at the clinic. To the mix, Dr. Frick added a monetary goal around which her troops could rally. Based on annual profit goals, her aim was to produce a higher percentage of profit yearly. Progress was tracked on an illustrated thermometer placed on a wall visible only to the staff.

The game worked! One year, the annual reward found the group in Las Vegas, having a wonderful time together.

On the other hand, not making the stated target goal, even if short by only $200, meant going nowhere.

"We liked it, and we liked Dr. Ava. We realized that here was a brilliant person who was *really* good at what she did. And innovative. She was into Standard Process and Nutraceuticals for her animals long before other veterinarians. When, later, she expanded to Animal Chiropractic, it was because she wanted to help the animals more."

Even rats.

"One day, a woman showed up at Pet Station with a female white rat. Her story was that they had gotten her for their boys, six and eight, but lately, she had started biting them. The family had decided to have her euthanized. While they lived in Washington, the town seven miles to the north of Union, and their veterinarian was in that town, he had told her he was not sure how to handle a rat and suggested she bring her to Union for that.

"I got the drift right away. Boys at that age can be fast-moving and not necessarily always full of patience and compassion, and rats are kind of like mules: they only take abuse once. What happens to them is recorded and remembered FOREVER. Your turn will come is the idea.

"Well, the boys attempted teasing her a second time and were met with a different result, so here she was, looking to me like a perfectly good rat.

"I had never had a pet rat and wasn't sure that was my intent now, but she didn't deserve to die. So, I asked the woman two questions: first, was it alright for me to find her a new home and not bump her off? That was agreeable. And, second, what was her name?

"'Minnie,' I was told. Well, maybe that was part of the problem because Minnie was a mouse name!

"With a roll of the tongue (not common in rural Missouri), I named her 'Reba Rat.' And, you guessed it, my clinic was her new home.

"We all enjoyed our days together. Reba lived at the clinic (a common thread with animals belonging to a veterinarian). When I had children come in with their parents, I would go get her. My hair was shoulder-length, and she would hide around my neck, only her tail partially exposed, flicking periodically, flipping my hair as it did. The game here was waiting to see how long it took one of the kids to notice and then say something about my hair movement. Then, I would take her off my shoulders and let them pet her. Afterward, slipping Reba into my white coat pocket, where she would occasionally peek out, quickly allowed her to retreat back to safety.

"When my Gramme suffered a stroke and was in the hospital, knowing she had

spent many years on a farm tending animals, I believed that if I exposed her to any animal, it would help her recover. Plus, there was no way her cat, Missie Peeker, would be happy finding herself in a hospital room. Getting a dog past the nurse station would be a challenge, but, I thought, Reba could be just the ticket! I could hide her in a duffle bag and not have to worry about any noise. Perfect!

"*Reba and I headed to the hospital. I got in to Grammie's room and told her it was me. At first, she was mumbling and not making much sense. So, I took Reba out and told her I had brought my pet rat to visit her. I put Reba down next to her, and Grammie started to pet her, stroking her gently.*

"*Then she asked, 'What happened to kitty's tail?'*

"*At that moment, I knew undoubtedly that Grammie knew it was me. She knew that cats and I went together. So, if it was a little fluffy thing, it must be a kitten. And kittens have fluffy tails.*

"*I reiterated that this was a rat, not a kitten. That is why the tail feels funny. Rats have a furless tail.*

"*About that time, a nurse opened the door, and I start thinking I have been caught. But, she came in and took vitals and didn't say a word.*

*"Not 15 minutes later, the doctor
shows up. Oh great, I think. But, he
commences telling me about his roommate
in med school, who had a pet rat in their
apartment. Wow! I had taken the chance
that I would have to ask for forgiveness as
opposed to taking one to get permission.
Either way, it was a chance I took, and
nothing came of it, except a moment of
therapy that day for my Grammie and
proof that animals help heal.*

*"Reba and I packed up, and she was
returned back to her space. Grammie had
a full recovery.*

*"Reba lived beyond the typical
lifespan of a rat, despite twice undergoing
surgery for a mammary tumor. Eventually,
it made its way into her lungs, but by then,
she was four and had lived a long,
beautiful rat life!*

Events at the clinic continued to bring new and
humorous adventures almost daily.

*"Along about early 1995, a client
couple comes in to work one Saturday
morning, distressed about the fact that they
had found seven baby skunks in their barn
in an unused stall. Earlier that week, a
skunk had been killed on their gravel road,
and their assumption was that she was the
mother. The babies had gotten so hungry
the couple became aware of their
movements.*

"Sure enough, they all were less than two weeks old, judging by their eyes still being closed, and all up for grabs.

" 'Sure, I'll take them,' I piped up. I had never been close to a skunk, and this sounded like a fun opportunity to learn about them. To that point, I had not calculated how much money I would soon spend payin' employees to help me care for and clean up after them.

"What I did learn was that skunks do not have any mean bones in their bodies. They are loveable and playful. No two are marked alike, and, though they will puff up, they do not become offensive until after three to four months. Topping that, if you pick one up while quickly scooping their tail under their bottom, they don't spray.

"Bless my heart, all seven lived on, which, for wild animals in captivity, I took as a tremendous complement to our care and attention to their innate needs.

"As they neared three months, they began eatin' cat food ... each fighting the others for their share of the grub, gettin' their feet totally immersed in the bowl and then leaving footprints on the cement floor of the kennel area at the clinic where they were now housed.

"Jodi, our kennel attendant, hosed down their breakfast mess every time, after which she ran a dry rag mop over the floor *to prevent slipping by other staff members. And two skunks took this to be like a ride at the county fair. They fought over riding rights on the rag mop, pushing each other off like some 'king of the hill' game, the victor takin' the pole position and hanging on as Jodi swayed the mophead back and forth across the floor.*

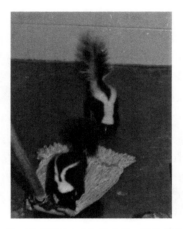

Skunk riding a rag mop & one in the que!

"I took a video of this and sent it to "America's Funniest Home Videos," but never heard back.

"Setting that humor aside, the real skunk story involves a visit I made to Cedarcrest Manor, the senior residency and nursing home in Washington, Missouri.

"From time to time, I had done animal visits to the place, always with dogs. One day, I selected the three most friendly

skunks to take on a trip with Keoki, Joey, and myself. Once inside, most of the residents took the typical keep-back approach, except one petite, elderly woman, who had come in escorted by her daughter, (herself in her sixties), wearing a navy-blue-and-white-polka-dot dress fringed with a small, rounded-lace collar and belted at the waist—a beautiful church dress.

"When this woman saw the skunks, she lit up. Her eyes beamed, and she wanted desperately to hold one.

"Doing my due diligence, I had restricted their morning meal and made sure they had plenty of time to play and potty. However, with animals, as Johnny Carson could have attested to quickly, being from Nebraska, there are no guarantees.

"I looked at her daughter and explained the situation since her mother was begging to let her hold one. Returning my message with a reticent smile, the daughter nodded approvingly.

"I found a towel to put on the resident's lap, just in case, and, picking the one I considered the sweetest, I handed her over.

"In that precious moment, I understood why she needed to hold a little, warm animal one more time. She, too, as

*the daughter shared with me, had grown
up on a farm and loved animals.*

*"The little skunk had crawled up next
to her neck and just lay there as she was
petted and stroked. The look on the
woman's face was of complete satisfaction,
perhaps from memories of her past animal
relationships. To touch and hold a young
animal again with the affection that only
one who really loves them could exude,
made her life come full circle.*

*"A moment in time given, a wish
fulfilled, I left Cedarcrest Manor that day
with a larger heart than the one with which
I had entered. In giving, I had received in
abundance. Never will I forget that look in
her eyes and the smile painted across her
face. Priceless."*

* * *

The circle of Life turned for the better in Frick's
personal life, too. In March of 1996, a healthy baby boy
arrived, whom Ava and Tony named 'Dalton Eli Kuenzel."

*"While I had done some babysitting
during high school, none were with infants,
and we had no family with babies. So, my
reality of newborns was limited to animals.*

(Go figure, right?)

*"One night, before any ultrasound
was done, I woke from the funniest dream.
In the dream, I have delivered the baby.
The nurses checking it over exclaim as
they are looking at the baby's feet and*

toes, 'It's a boy, and he's an orange tabby.
He's going to be fluffy, too!'

"See, the long tufts between the toes
are a harbinger of the kind of fur a cat will
have. A mantra of mine is that you cannot
beat an orange tabby. They typically have
great personalities. And it has proven the
same for my son, too!

The arrival of their son changed forever how Dr. Frick looked at and acted toward her professional practice and career. The blessed event was also the bellwether of a gathering storm that, given a little more time, would swamp Ava's marriage to Tony.

To this time, Dr. Frick had been by-the-book traditional in her approach to her Veterinary practice. Surgery, dental, x-rays, IVs, drugs, you name it … she dispensed the expected norm of her medicines like everyone else. Changing that routine never had entered her mind, even as a thought. But, now her outlook was different.

"… I was turning 40 and having a
child in my life. I began to look at life
differently."

From her new perspective, she realized, probably for one of the first times, that she had not accomplished what she had achieved with animals all by herself. She could see there were people to thank.

Her son's birth brought changes to her time and schedule at work, too. Emergency calls at night were cut off. She had needed more sleep weeks before his arrival, and for weeks after still more was necessary. In her absence, relief veterinarians maintained the sizeable client workload she had created, assisted by the visible support of her well-trained, flexible staff. Both the clinic and staff came a long way from their rough-and-tumble early days.

Of course, the primary concern remained the welfare of the animals, but Dr. Frick's view of the practice was more matter-of-fact now.

> *"This particular day, I had the*
> *common Dachshund patient come in—*
> *unable to navigate because of*
> *intervertebral disc disease. My frustration*
> *set in, and I said to the dog, 'I can give you*
> *some drugs, but I can't fix your problem.'*
> *That day, I realized I had to learn about*
> *other ways to help the animals more."*

* * *

Because of that Dachshund, in the following year, Frick invested her precious free time into trips to Hillsdale, Illinois, for one week every month for six months to get certified to offer Animal Chiropractic services. As was her wont all her life, she made the sacrifice thinking about how it would provide more care for the animals under her supervision. And, no doubt, for the growing boy living under her wing and rooftop.

Candidates for certification must hold a Doctor of Chiropractic or Doctor of Veterinary Medicine degree. Passing a comprehensive written exam and completing an intensive, practical-skills review is part of the enrollment process. Dr. Frick easily certified and received her American Veterinary Chiropractic Association (AVCA) certification, a status valid for a period of three years, after which re-certification was a requirement.

> *"The chiropractic training was very*
> *intense, and we were taught to see with our*
> *fingertips. Palpation became a tender*

process motioning every single vertebral
segment or extremity joint. Visually
imagining what was happening beneath
the skin and muscle surface. This was a
new way of listening. Through it, I became
very 'in tune' with the animal I was
working on.

* * *

By August of 1997, having completed her animal-chiropractic basics, Frick continued to take advanced training from 1998 to 2004 by participating in an ongoing program called Options for Animals. Already a practicing DVM with a loyal following and a growing reputation among her peers, she continued to expand her know-how, responsibilities, and control skills. Again, she pushed herself beyond normal limits, knowing that taking on each new field made her a novice practitioner in that new area, though one with an immense and growing passion for doing more and more for animals she knew experienced pains and soreness.

As she pushed herself in her profession, she may have been pushing herself out of her marriage. Frick's personal life seemed to be tracking more like a roller-coaster than a rocket ride to the stars. Tony and she did not see eye to eye enough to carry on together. When they blinked, Dalton found himself living in a household managed solely by his mother.

With that phase of her life completed and hope for a newer, brighter future ahead of her, Frick moved herself and her son to a Germantown Road location near Washington, Missouri, into a suitable log-cabin house where she and Dalton could make their home. Her private world had not wholly turned upside down, because Tony and Ava agreed to maintain effective communication with each other for the sake of their only child, an arrangement that worked out.

Already at one of her lowest ebbs with her marriage days turned for the worst, Frick's discovery by chance of a golden nugget of hope lead her to want to reach out again, to expand not only herself but also her practice to a whole new level of understanding and applied technology, as well as a new company connection. Her keen desire to help led her to Standard Process, Inc., the whole-foods supplement company started by Dr. Royal Lee almost 90 years earlier.

Frick's newly formed contact's philosophy of care aligned well with her own, as stated by the company's owners:

"Healthy Soil. Healthy Plants. Healthy Lives. Standard Process has been dedicated to making high-quality and nutrient-dense therapeutic supplements for three generations. We focus on achieving holistic health through nutrition. From our organic, regenerative farming practice to our Nutrition Innovation Center research facility, we are committed to clinical science that advances health and changes lives. From soil to supplement, there is a direct relationship between the earth, what you consume, and your overall well-being."

Her new connection motivated Frick to develop an operational tool to advance and better target the nutritional needs of dogs and cats. She created the Clinical Animal Nutrition Survey (CAN survey), a benchmark innovation.

Once again, Frick was working at the forefront of her industry; no one before her had worked out such a survey for animals. Having seen the problems of working without this needed tool directly, she did her usual and invented something useful that did not exist, for which there was a demonstrated need. A testimonial to the nature of her research ethic, the tool is still in use today.

Once again, she had burned the midnight oil … this time, after putting her young son to bed night after night.

While work engulfed most of her days, here and there she got in some horseback-riding and an occasional country-western dance; that is, when not spending precious time with her gregarious and growing son. The balancing act seemed to be working because opportunity came knocking.

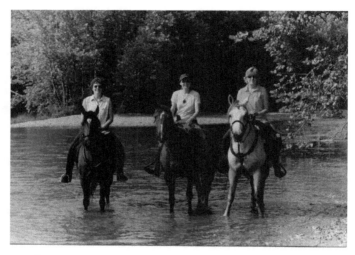

Lanie – Iris – Ava astride horses at Cross Country Trail Ride in Eminence, Missouri.

BioScan in New Mexico produced equine shin pads based on a unique approach involving the use of lasers. Since their product protected the hocks of horses, and Dr. Frick's clinical reputation was widespread, they caught each other's attention. The company's laser-based concept got Frick to thinking about using full-level laser devices in an improved way for different animal species. Once again true to her artistic and innovative leanings, she contacted Nadine M. Donahue, president of BioScan, and asked if she would mind Frick developing improved pads with diodes planned and correctly placed for use with horses and other types of animals' backs.

Nadine had no objection; in fact, she welcomed Frick's input so much that she eventually manufactured new "Laser Spinal Pads" (as Frick had called them). Sadly, Frick never thought of applying for a patent; though, she did take some pleasure in knowing that she had been the first to develop such a product. One could say easily and with authority that "Ava Frick was using lasers before lasers were cool!"

The new Laser Spinal Pads launched with success in 1998. The concept of them was easy for practitioners to understand: the laser-light diodes presented differing wavelengths aimed at screened areas of a spine, enabling more mobility and correction. The product worked well.

Today, similar products are on the market but not the originals. Somehow, in a mysterious manner, the original plates for the pads were lost, and the BioScan company was sold to Revita-Patch. Frick did receive some royalties in the early years of her product's sales, but because she had failed to take out a patent, her cut was somewhat of a pyrrhic victory.

By the time all connections to the first product evaporated, Frick had moved on already. Always inquisitive and growing in her purpose to offer as much help for animals as possible, she discovered yet another technology that, by now, she considered more advanced and possibly the wave of the future in animal rehabilitative care.

At home, Frick was starting to find in her boy a good companion just about the time he turned three. They celebrated his birthday, along with another new arrival.

> *" 'Chuckie' came to live with us when Dalton was three. He was a miniature horse, not a dwarf. He looked like a pony, was 33 years old, and had raised many, many kids over the years. It was time for him to retire and only work part-time. The*

arrangement was that we would not 'own' him but could have him if we took care of him. That would not be a problem. And they knew that, too. Chuckie and Dalton were 'best buds' from the get-go. He allowed Dalton to learn how to have fun controlling something. Chuckie would not be telling him what to do or how to do it.

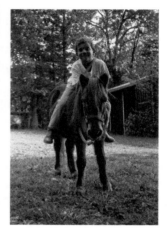

Dalton and Chuckie.

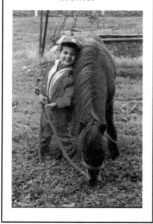

The Day Chuckie Came Home.

"Like most boys, Dalton enjoyed speed, and for a few years, Chuckie was happy to accommodate him in short spurts. Chuckie shared his knowledge, and Dalton learned how to ride. He was gentle, calm, understanding, and yet managed his space with dignity. For the first year, I lead Dalton around. By the time he was four, he was 'chomping at the bit' to ride by himself. This particular day I am

gardening and agreed that he could solo ride, with a few restrictions. Mainly stay in the yard. I am not sure what he had been doing, but at this moment, he and Chuckie are running full speed around the corner of the house.

"My first knee-jerk reaction is a result of my past pony incident. Thinking the worst, I go into a rant of one thing after another that he should not be doing. Then I look at Dalton's face, and it is beaming! He looks directly at me, with full conviction, slams his little hand down on top of the saddle horn and says, 'Don't worry, Mom, I can whoa him!' That was the last time I ever attempted to inflict any of my fears upon my son. It was totally unfair of me to put him into my 'box.' He went on to excel at riding, tricks, and otherwise using some deep-seated innate Native American heritage (inherited from his Dad) to become one with a horse.

"Later that year, we come home from work one night, and Chuckie is drooling; head drooped, he does not look good. I have no idea how long he has been this way, other than he was fine in the morning. Common for old horses is that as the teeth wear, they have difficulty chewing grass and hay. It is my suspicion that he is choking. I immediately call a horse veterinarian I knew was not too far away. Dr. Roth arrives and does all that she could, but the mass would not budge. So, at 9 PM, we load him up into the trailer

and head north to a hospital for help.
Praying that he is still alive when we get
there. Along the way, Dalton looks at me
very seriously and says, 'If Chuckie dies, I
will cry.' And I replied, 'If Chuckie dies, I
will cry too, Dalton.' He did not die. After
two days in the hospital, he was ready to
come home. We altered his food, got used
to seeing what we called 'Chuckie wads'
on the ground or floating in the water
trough, and enjoyed him for nine more
years, sharing many fun moments and
great rides. They were such a cute pair. I
said a tearful good-bye to him at 42, seven
years later. I don't remember, however,
when we had the back-hoe guy dig a trench
with a graduated walkway for the
traditional equine vet to come out and put
Chuckie to sleep. We had wanted it to be
as easy as possible for him. The back-hoe
driver, I do remember, returned to cover
the hillside with him at the bottom before
Dalton got home from school that day.

"Happy trails, Chuckie!"

* * *

Up to 1999, Ava's core of attention had centered around

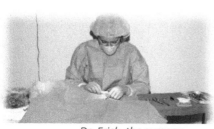

Dr. Frick, the surgeon

animals, not humans. Aside from a few close friendships, her daily outlook for her life had run good and bad—an assessment determined by and consistently dependent upon the conditions she observed of the animals in her care. This was tempered by what results she had been able to accomplish for each customer at any given time. In other words, her professional life and her personal life mirrored a roller-coaster ride. In her estimation, something needed to change.

Brushing aside notions of her having found Aladdin's lamp on some deserted beach—after all, she was landlocked in Missouri, one particular conversation she had with a person whom she did not particularly know, caught her by surprise and changed her general view of life significantly.

The person, a representative of an international non-profit group to which Frick already had a favorable leaning, had just asked her for a significant donation to their cause. Frick, in the process of considering what he had asked of her, and what she might want to do about it, had not made up her mind when, in counterpoint to his persuasive plea for help, she stated, *"I'm about animals. I donate to animal causes; I'm here for them. Others can worry about people."*

His answer floored her: "Ava, if we don't help the people of Earth, the animals don't stand a chance."

His logic was simple and direct. And so persuasive. The dichotomy of people versus animals in her past had goaded Frick to move past the status quo and to be an unstoppable force in her chosen profession, but his simple statement in reply to her cherished view won her over. Her subsequent outpourings of help, in turn, motivated and shaped the future nature of the way she worked. Her new outlook toward all living creatures included humans from that point forward. In her process of change, she gained a unique perspective from which she could be more herself—one quite different from her early years.

> *"That man who got me to make the
> donation changed me. He shifted my view
> about people. It was like my life flipped*

from animals first to humans first. I've looked at life differently than I did in my childhood ever since then ... not that it was the only turning point because the birth of my son Dalton three years earlier certainly started the process. For me, at 44, the value of humans, and my care level for them, for the first time, went beyond my love of animals. I had flipped into the alignment of living among other people, and I have felt comfortable with it ever since."

Perhaps, that change in her life came at the most opportune time for her. Unknown to her, then, it would not be long before she met someone with an extensive background and long stretch of years in another, unrelated field involving athletes, specifically baseball. This new connection would lead her to an opportunity to become a critical vocal advocate for all of her peer doctors. Dr. Frick, at last, was about to come full circle with her real valuation to herself and to others.

"When I was young, I had patience. I learned that from the need to wait on the kittens. Along the way, when confronted with my desire to attain my veterinarian status, and others confronted me with votes of no-confidence such as, 'It's not likely;' 'You won't be able to do it' (euthanasia); 'It won't happen; it's a man's profession, and very few women ever get in;' 'It's tough, it will be eight, long years of college, et cetera, I chose tenacity over patience. I was about getting what I went after. My approach for that part of my life bled over to all the other parts as well. In

that, the time for patience had died,
replaced by a determination to come out
on top of success on my terms."

* * *

CHAPTER 8: FITNESS IN MOTION

Ava consulted her staff when it became apparent in 2000, that there was more that she could do for animals by stepping outside of her customary traditional approach (i.e., diagnoses, surgeries, and drugs) to her veterinary practice at Pet Station. Part of the new idea she floated would be to take some local property and convert it into a rehabilitation facility for animals—the logical next step to integrating what she had been soaking up the past three years to give it back to her community.

"I was enjoying this new education. My eyes were opened to new opportunities, and my mind was loving it. I was in my element. My holdfast to traditional veterinary medicine was surgery. I enjoyed surgery and was very good at it. I had gotten 30-pound dog spays down to a flawless seven minutes. Then one day, as I completed closing the abdomen and burying all sutures, so there was nothing to bother the dog, there was nothing left for me. Laying the forceps and needle holders down on the instrument tray, I looked up and said to myself, 'I have done enough. This game is over. Time to sell and move on.'"

That decision was an epiphany for Dr. Frick. It would lead her to the "bamboo door" of a new opportunity, even as the "iron door" closed. It would take her to a widening of her sphere of influence in her chosen field and beyond its current scope; in fact, it would take her afield almost to the doorstep of her favorite baseball team, the St. Louis Cardinals.

Gene Gieselmann, for a multi-decade span of time, had been the Athletic Trainer for the Cardinals. There, he rubbed elbows with the likes of Hall of Famers Lou Brock and Bob Gibson, among other greats of the game. In 1999, Gieselmann, retired from the world of baseball, intending to move on to his next professional venue, veterinary medicine and health care for animals. His purpose led him straight to Dr. Frick in a roundabout way.

Having researched and read about her in recent years, Gieselmann understood that she was more than merely at the forefront of her field; she was ahead of her time. Prior to learning of her animal-oriented methodology, the only hydro-therapy he knew was that used on professional athletes, including underwater treadmills used by one of the two Chicago teams. To Gieselmann, anyone using that innovative rehabilitative therapy in another field, especially with animals, rightfully should be positioned as well ahead of her time. This made Dr. Frick a real candidate to work with, in his view.

Prior to Gieselmann and Frick finding each other, lawmakers in Missouri mandated a law that any animal-rehab clinic must have a certified veterinarian on-site or one intimately connected to their business. This wrinkle—the bill would later be batted about in the capital, Jefferson City, and vetoed by the governor but not before being waged against by Gieselmann and Frick's side-by-side testimony in front of the legislatures of the Missouri Senate and House in 2003-2004—would force Gieselmann to have to hire (at extra expense) a full-time veterinarian for his facility.

It was a "Catch-22" situation for him; he was damned if he did and damned if he didn't. In answer to the potential problem, he chose to pursue and establish a connection with Dr. Frick to help him knock out this legal requirement. And he initially did so despite several damning admonishments voiced at him from medical doctors he knew to not work with her since she was not only "not their kind of doctor" but, worse, a known, outspoken animal chiropractor and veterinarian. As a result, Gieselmann and Frick became not only professional allies connected to his Animal Rehab Foundation (ARF!) but also long-term friends.

While they were in some negotiations to create a business together, Gieselmann, having decided to follow other friends' recommendations to obtain as many allies as he could muster, approached the University of Missouri College of Veterinary Medicine, Frick's Alma Mater. Because of her complementary practice style, they were opposed to giving him their seal of approval if Frick was a partner. Choosing to align with the university, he asked for names of veterinarians that they would recommend fulfilling the state's requirement for him to have one full-time on his staff. Unfortunately, none of their recommended graduates had animal rehabilitation skills, limiting the appeal of his services. Within six months, unfortunately, the first veterinarian hired moved on, and the second, though he was a great guy, lacked sufficient skill and physiotherapy training to pull in more business by appropriately treating this type of patient.

Making matters more difficult for Gieselmann, over the course of the next year, the Vet School only referred 24 cases to his facility—hardly enough to keep the ARF! doors open. Eventually, he reached out again to Dr. Frick, who, by now, had her new Animal Fitness Center (AFC) facility ramped up. (She had opened AFC in March 2002. Gieselmann opened his facility in Fenton, Missouri, in April 2002.)

Based on their friendship and her assessment of his predicament, Dr. Frick agreed to help him. Frick volunteered time to ARF! two to three times a week—in itself a significant boost to Gieselmann's fledgling business.

Because of her contributions derived from her knowledge of animal nutrition and, of course, her many years of experience in this business arena, Gieselmann extended his run beyond everyone's initial expectations, par for the course within Frick's professional life and sphere of influence. On average, rehabilitated dogs treated under Frick's care lived to 16-17 years of age without a measurable decline in their quality of living. In other words, Dr. Frick could be considered by some a "miracle worker."

Gieselmann recalls some animals, like the Jack Russell breed dog who by licking his paws developed various cancers after he ran through his owners' chemical-laden, green lawns.

"Ava was a 'smart cookie' when it came to her four-legged 'children,'" noted Gieselmann, "... because she practiced what a lot of other veterinarians did not. Indeed, we both used Eastern medicines and Standard Process products, even acupuncture, for the benefit of our animals."

Gieselmann watched as Frick's treatment of one animal after another caused them to get better, including a dog named "Gus" who had been laid out on a stretcher, unable to walk at all, yet that same day walked out of the clinic. On leaving, Gus left behind a hamper full of dampened staff handkerchiefs, as well as teardrop trails of joy across his clinic's floor.

Gieselmann, despite his best intentions, moved to close his clinic for economic reasons after (too late) asking for and getting sound financial advice from Frick to rein in costs and make the clinic spend less than it earned. He had, in his words, "...gotten over my ski tops."

Meanwhile, in Dr. Frick's hands, scores of animals continued to depart from her clinic, time and again, with their owners thrilled about the immediate changes they saw and exhilarated by their renewed expectations for their pets to live out their lives in good health for years to come.

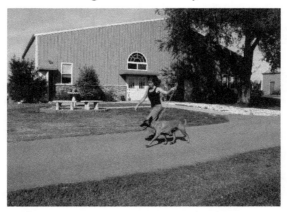

Animal Fitness Center, client and her dog

* * *

Two years earlier, in 2000, Frick had embraced microcurrent electrical therapy (MET), which had an immediate and positive effect on her career and results. Her initial interest in the possibilities of Alpha-Stim® technology (AST) led her well beyond the horizons of even her own expectations, but there was an exciting, earlier beginning to this chapter of her life.

Coincident with her college days as undergraduate, other researchers looked into the use of cranial electrotherapy stimulation (CES) as a means to assist animals' dispositions and to rehabilitate certain body conditions. Dr. Daniel Kirsch, a Ph.D. in neurobiology, was a leading proponent of the technology. In part, Kirsch's involvement came about because he wanted to know more about animals; conversely, he noted that animal professionals had not yet profoundly embraced human therapies, not having been trained in those fields. However, because of their extensive study of animals, they could be counted upon to have empathy and affinity for those displaying non-optimum conditions, coupled with a desire to help them return to better days health-wise. Any initial lack of active interest in the AST technology was not because they were not bright enough to handle the extra data load or to understand the subject; they were, simply put, not as keenly focused on people as with animals. In Dr. Frick, Kirsch believed he found someone adept at both. Meeting her for the first time, he realized she was a DVM not only capable of grasping the efficacy of AST for both humans and animals but also possessing a genuine interest in learning all about it.

"Ava was a leader, not your typical blue-collar doctor acting more like a technician, using only what they were taught, and no more, and then moving on to the next patient. She seemed a leader—someone whose natural interest moved beyond what was on the table in front of her and toward innovators in her field of endeavor and their products. While she was an excellent clinician and a noted 'horse whisperer,' she also excelled at understanding the science of what we were about in our field."

The trouble with bright doctors, even those with more than a passing interest in scientific innovations, was that most of them did not operate well within corporate settings. And Dr. Frick, according to Kirsch, fell in that category of doctor—a bit hard to work with inside of corporate offices but brilliant in her natural environment; and gifted within a versatile, broad scope of activities.

Kirsch came to his career in neurobiology from an interest in the bio-physics arena of study and application, whereas Frick arrived at hers by studying physical therapy in a way that her curiosity urged her to go beyond limits that other doctors set for themselves. When other Vet-Med graduates were content to operate as clinicians maintaining the status quo, Frick's experiences moved her gradually toward this other science and its potentials, bolstered by her abiding interest to help other species of living creatures. She was, in other words, willing to change and move beyond the time she lived in, motivated by that purpose.

The secret of AST, according to Kirsch, is that it is derived from vitalistic philosophy—(Vitalism, school of scientific thought—the germ of which dates from Aristotle—that attempts … to explain the nature of life as resulting from a vital force peculiar to living organisms and different from all other effects found outside living things. Source: Britannica.com)—the basis of all religions and all healthcare systems, except Western medicine, which limits us to being the sum of our parts. Other systems recognize a separate life-force as part of our anatomy. Acupuncture is the best-known example. This force can be thought of as a polarized electrical field running along specific paths in the body that, when altered, can result in disease or health. The Chinese speak of this bioelectricity as "ch'i;" East Indians call it "Prana."

What was unusual, in Kirsch's view, about Frick, fortuitously so, was that she keenly grasped right away not only the potential of the AST technology but also how its application might benefit animals; in that regard, she moved well past the known clinical parameters of the time.

Armed with her newly won expertise, Frick shortly was invited to accept a position with the company as Veterinary Medical Director as well as in the field, where she acted as a product distributor wholly capable of explaining AST products and the beneficial effects of their correct usage. In doing so, she performed under the aegis of a company division that she, in fact, had helped create along with Kirsch.

If Kirsch and Frick were talking to brick walls, at first, it was because of finding themselves up against the myopic approach to the education of doctors that formalized medicine adopted long ago. Nascent, inquiring minds filled with honest curiosity expressed by young Med students new to the disciplines of their science were being stifled. Kirsch called out the oppressiveness of what he termed "N2D2 Medicine"—meaning name the diagnosis to name the drug—and politely aimed a middle finger at the resultant robotic mentality of medical-school students who were graduated void of any active interest in what could be the cutting edge of medicine or potential fodder for the growth and well-being of their minds beyond expecting paychecks from the clinic and babies from home.

The majority of DVMs, at the time, graduated to expect themselves at work in private practices supported only by a small number of employed assistants; aside from a much smaller, select group going on to specialize in research and/or teach at universities. That widespread attitude among most veterinary-medicine practitioners did give rise, eventually, to a bell-curve line of expansion in the industry. However, Millennials, for the most part, shifted toward steady employment inside corporate-owned animal hospitals employing as many as 25 doctors and 100 assistants—cogs in a new giant wheel that guaranteed paychecks accompanied by vacations, insurance coverage, and other perks, not to mention meaty profits for corporate shareholders, possibly at the expense of the best model of healthcare for the animals they saw and treated.

Kirsch, on the other hand, found that Dr. Frick lived, breathed, and thought at a wholly different level of intellectuality and understanding. She capably duplicated what he taught her and actively explored applications of the data she had learned well beyond even *his* "norm." This innovative attitude got her wondering about saving more horses and how this might be accomplished through Alpha-Stim and its related products. In other words, her fledgling personal interest in AST, fueled by her caring attitude to help her own patients, had not only led her to the science of microcurrents but also helped her marshal in new applications with it.

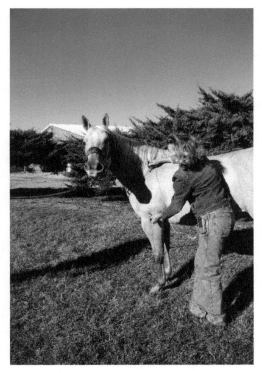

Barbie gets Alpha-Stim Treatment

Dr. Frick, by now, had bridged the gap between running a daily practice at her clinic and pushing her personal evolution out far enough to create an attention span of keen interest in yet another scientific field. Her use of the technology advanced beyond even one of its leading proponent's (Kirsch) expectations at the time. Furthermore, she exhibited great patience, a rare quality among innovators, while desirous of giving people more help than what they had expected for their animals. Doing that often meant having to go off the clock of work-time management, producing a positive effect upon Dr. Kirsch, who said about her, "I love healers … people who care enough. I like doctors who are interested in life, who stay up nights seeking answers, who look for ways to improve the 'vibes' coming from animals (and humans). I love those people, and Ava Frick is one of those."

Veterinary students who let themselves get abused by professors with the "right answers"—the blind leading the blind, end up as low self-esteem, semi-professional, blue-collar clinicians. Not so, Dr. Frick. From the get-go, with AST, she was unusually comfortable talking with important MDs as she ably showed them how the newest technology products worked and, importantly, in their view, how using Alpha-Stim could save or earn them more money. However, that was not her boundary line. With her natural gifts of intuition and vision, she not only merely envisioned applications for different animal species but also the need for correct dosages for a specific situation or conditions—a mammoth task for which she took the time to develop and codify, thereby setting an industry standard that is followed by others to this day.

Under the aegis of Dr. Kirsch, Dr. Frick lectured at the American Academy of Pain Management. Kirsch has had several articles published in PPM – *Practical Pain Management* magazine. He also holds a seat today on its editorial board.

Today, a recurrent mutual interest the two doctors have is the possible application of AST to the burgeoning problems associated with fentanyl and oxycontin opioid addictions and their effects; and, of course, more usages applicable to animals. There may even be a window of opportunity for psychiatrists to drop their use of abusive and brain-damaging ECT (electric shock) "treatments" altogether. Curbing that would be a boon for humanity and real sanity. (Imagine repeated doses of 400 or more watts of pure electricity coursing through your brain! Would you want that?! Real human beings across a wide range of ages that includes infants currently endure such torture today.)

Both Drs. Frick and Kirsch agree that doctors who really care, who have an interest in helping others, do find that their patients, human and animal, like and prefer getting well and, in so many ways, they let them know it.

Interestingly, surveys show, doctors who keep an active interest in their work also experience reduced levels of personal stress—an evident and common denominator shared readily by Drs. Frick and Kirsch. One could even postulate a working formula for an individual health and success regimen that would benefit any doctor, starting with: Pay attention to your patients and create your interest in them continuously.

* * *

The middle of the first decade of the 21st Century was the commencement of a busy time for the good Dr. Frick. She received the Hartz Mountain Veterinarian of the Year Runner-Up award given to veterinarians who demonstrated outstanding commitment to patients and their families and their communities. A year later, she published her first book, *Fitness in Motion: Keeping Your Equine's Zones at Peak Performance,* brought out by the prestigious publisher Lyons Press. With that caché added to her reputation, she accepted many offers to "take her show on the road."

Additionally, she accepted the responsible position of Complementary Section Chairman for the American Veterinary Medical Association annual conferences. That meant she had to secure topics and presenters for the five-day meetings. She hosted a radio talk show out of Tempe, Arizona, *Animal Attraction,* while simultaneously raising her son, taking horse trips (some with and some without him), and learning what it meant to be a "wrestling mom."

In 1989, Frick joined Kiwanis Club International, a nonprofit group that began in 1915, which brought her in touch with Rich Sandoval, the former high-school principal during Lanie's tenure there. By 2008, she was serving as President of the Union Kiwanis Club. Because outside of club meetings Sandoval and Frick ran busy schedules, contact between them remained confined to club-related activities.

Sandoval established his opinion of Frick almost from the start. He recognized her diligence as a hard worker who was creative and, importantly to him, well-organized. Their mutual interest in recruiting qualified members to the club revealed to him that she could come up with novel recruitment schemes, including scripted videos.

Before Dr. Frick's clinic and busy business schedule expanded too much for her to continue to be very active with the Kiwanis club, she also worked with Sandoval and other members on seasonal activities like the annual Christmas-stocking events. In 2007, she volunteered her valuable horse trailer as a sled to carry a large number of gifts intended to be delivered to local children. With unloading done by other volunteers, Sandoval and Frick sat and talked, rambling on and reminiscing about a variety of subjects, including her (then) 11-year-old son Dalton.

According to Sandoval, Ava was "driven" by her professional interests, and she expected a lot from others. He surmised that several men likely had an interest in her over the years but might have found it hard to meet up to her expectations.

Well, amen! Most real professionals do expect a lot of their peers. And Frick was right to expect of others at least as much as she was capable of demanding from and producing herself.

Once in a blue moon, though, Ava Frick would still let her hair down out on the open plains along Highway 100 outside of Ballwin, Missouri. There, a particular country-western bar was the favorite place to be in off-hours after work.

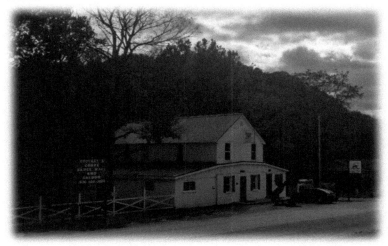

Stovall's C&W music hall

An authentic, historic honky-tonk music hall housed in a white building replete with a statue of a horse rearing up on the front lawn, the place featured national and local, award-winning, live-music-talent shows on Friday and Saturday nights, and an open-mic on Wednesdays. The site came replete with couples and line dancing offered every night, tasty monthly barbecues, a full liquor bar, and seasonal campfires situated under the leaves of a tree-lined grove outback. Located in Wildwood in West St. Louis County, the venue doubled as a watering hole and party hall for birthdays, reunions, bridal showers, holiday and family get-togethers, nights out with friends, retirements, and weddings. Their slogan is still one of the best around those parts:

"Our beer is cold and music sizzling hot. Grab your posse, swing your honey, scoot your boots, and Giddyup at Stovall's!"

Meanwhile, back at the ranch (circa 2009) ... the nation's economic downturn continued to impose stresses on Dr. Frick's business, the Animal Fitness Center at 1841 Denmark Road in Union since the meltdown was causing a domino effect. Small-business owners had to watch closely their P's and Q's.

Life as usual, of course, continued on. Entertainment for Frick still included dancing, horseback riding, and, for a while, Dalton's team roping. To support his activity at home, he and his Mom got a few cattle and built a roping arena, where she could watch him grow with her help.

In 2010, Dalton commenced high-school, and Dr. Frick published for the second time in the *Journal for Equine Veterinary Science*. Her article titled, "Horse Stretching Exercises; Are They Effective?" revealed her passion for horses publicly. For her, the momentous opportunity translated into yet another avenue to advance not only her pleasure and learning curve but also her knowledge, which she hoped would help others understand that magnificent animal more to the betterment of all horses and their owners.

A year later, in March, Dalton turned 15 and ushered in a new era of interest, another kind of horsepower: automotive. Not wanting to continue the work and effort they demanded, he was less interested in the four-legged variety. In that his Mom still harbored an active love for vehicle power and style, he was playing up to one of her affinities.

Ava, too, started to reassess aspects of her life and business. Expecting a new outcome from the same old activities of her past looked a bit insane to her. She understood that whatever had happened was done and gone, and if someone had to drive her future, she might as well be the one to take the wheel even if that meant driving on an uncharted road in all kinds of weather.

Even the weatherman could not accurately predict the changes that would alter the immediate future for Dalton and Ava. Suddenly, in a matter of minutes, most of Joplin, Missouri, was destroyed by a devastating tornado. Putting his primary interests on the backburner, like most Missourians, Dalton joined the front-runner Scientology Volunteer Ministers® (VMs) group and, backed by his Mom, spent the next five days of his life helping victims recover what sensibilities and cherished items they could from the demolished ruins. The process inspired Dalton. He discovered that helping people in dire need changed their outlooks and priorities well beyond previous expectations. The net effect was the tragedy brought them closer to each other. Good thing, too, because Dalton was about to embark on a quest that would require cheerleading from the stands, which Ava was more than willing to give.

Over the next three years of their lives, a lot of mutual involvement with wrestling took place throughout weekends and bunches of weeknights. Anticipating her son's needs, Ava thought *What better to get a guy in shape than a summer vacation boot-camp-style?*

> *"Dalton and I went to a boot camp*
> *about survival and team building. We*
> *spent two weeks out of the country on a*
> *ship in the ocean. The change of*
> *environment was good, but then I*
> *realized, watching him struggle through*

one of the group exercises in the water,
that Dalton didn't really know how to
swim! I felt like I had let him down. But
even more, I had let myself down as a
mother."

Back on dry land, wrestling matches continued. With Ava sitting in the bleachers as often as possible and urging her son on—his dad sat nearby on the sidelines, Dalton kept getting better and better at the sport, winning match after match under the guidance of his coaches.

* * *

By early 2012, Dr. Frick started thinking that she needed to move her business to the city. The economy had not rallied, and fewer people were willing to take off work for most of their day to make the long drive to Union. She ended up moving the clinic to Chesterfield and renaming it "Pet Rehab & Pain Clinic." (*"Pain was a better button."*) Now, instead of her walking two minutes to work—the clinic Dalton grew up in had been located on her farm—and her customers driving long distances, she was driving 50 minutes, one-way, every day, further stretching her time budget to its limit. But, she never looked or turned back.

"One trait in which I parallel Dad—
in addition to being tall and lean, blonde,
and gifted with his German facial
features—is that once we get an idea, and
decide to do it, it's too late to stop us."

This move was one of them. She had wanted to be in Eureka, but the place she had her eye on was leased. When her three-year lease neared renewal, she revisited Eureka, because Chesterfield already was expensive, and the lease contract was about to go up. Eureka, indeed, was available now! She initiated steps to get an agreement drawn up. With the legal rudiments in place, she refurbished a 1957 Shell Oil gasoline service station and moved the business into its present location at 105 East 5th Street.

Within a year, the horses were sold, and one of her favorite animals, Bobaloo, a donkey, was placed in a new home. Soon after, the two-horse trailers and the bright-red Ford F250 that had carried her and Dalton to many a horse-riding vacation or team-roping event across several states followed suit.

The sales marked the end of the old and the beginning of a new round of horizons of hope. Not all of their extra-curricular activities involved wrestlin', workin', hootin', and hollerin.'

Harkening back to her Kiwanis days, which ran simultaneously with her clinic expansions and letting her hair down at Stovall's, when paper-angel cutouts needed to be made and placed on the local Kiwanis' Christmas tree, Ava often was the creative brains for their designs. If puzzles needed coloring and assembly for the festivities that people would be happy at the related event, she and Dalton assembled them. They helped with decorations. They made stockings for gifts on her sewing machine, too. A proud Momma often looked over at her partner at the table, admiring how it was that she had raised a strong, independent, decent young man while doing research, writing articles, and building her company and reputation across an ever-widening sphere of influence.

When her first published book released, she was not only understandably proud of her two-year labor of love but also grateful for those who had helped her with the project: Barbara Hethcote her co-author, Randall Schilling her photographer, and her son Dalton, whose companionship and horse-exercise demonstrations with Chuckie added an intangible something unique to its pages.

Her life and career rolling faster now in 2013, the American Institute of Stress selected Dr. Frick as a Fellow and her human/animal-bond articles for *Combat Stress* and *Contentment* magazines published with success and approval.

Year after year, not only had her star continued to rise but also her son's wrestling skills. More than a decade after he began with the sport, a feat his Mom relishes to this day happened. She wrote and mailed out a letter about it to all of her family and to friends who had helped him throughout his life:

"Dalton Takes First in State Wrestling!

"Date: Sunday, 23 Feb 2014.

"While the Winter Olympics were celebrating the culmination of many medals, Missouri State High School Wrestling was awarding medals for the 'best of the best' wrestlers of the 2013 – 2014 season. Union High School is jumping up and down and screaming from the top of the school because Dalton Kuenzel took first place in the 182# Class 3 Championship! This is the first time Union took first in the state since 1991.

"Dalton has been a wrestler for 11 years. He began because his Dad enjoyed the sport and knew it was a character builder. Tony Kuenzel saw to it that Dalton made it to camps year-round. He knew champions only grew out of hours and hours of practice in learning all facets of this sport. Dalton had ups and downs over the years but continued to grow and develop wrestling moves that are his own and made this sport be unique to him and his style. And in his Senior year, Dalton has taken the school to the top, owning the podium on Saturday, February 22, 2014.

Dalton Wrestling

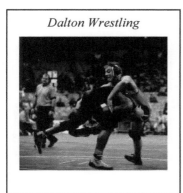

Dalton on Podium

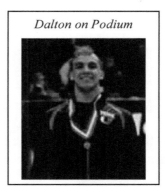

"His Mom revels in the young man he has become and the knowledge and skills he has gained. During each wrestling match over the years, her heart pounded, her emotions clenched, her life either raised or lowered momentarily by the win or loss. But this time, after the pounding heart and surge of emotions during Dalton's time on the mat, she cried tears for him, for his life, for this spectacular victory, for a dream come true—a dream Dalton created and followed through to the end by pure determination. Dalton is a champion in many ways, and now he's earned the title of 'Missouri State Wrestling Champion'!

"For those who have helped to bring Dalton along, wished him well, encouraged him in his endeavors, said

prayers over his life, nurtured his education, this win is also for you.

"For those who have helped his mother through the years to understand the mind of a boy, taught her what wrestling was about, helped with the critters so she could get out of town for a wrestling weekend, shared another great win or console over a loss, this win is also for you.

"Our hearts swell with emotion and thanksgiving to everyone who has been a part of Dalton's life and now also this success.

" Thank you eternally,

Dalton's Mother"

* * *

After high school, Dalton would not take to the idea of college. Though, as noted, a state-champion high-school wrestler, his interests turned more toward outdoor activities: fishing, hunting, working on his vehicles of necessity, and more volunteer work with the VMs, who show up immediately wherever help is needed after natural disasters and storms. Because of these self-determined interests and his will to help and serve others, his mother to this day never has missed the college diploma that (one day) may come, or not. On the contrary, she was (and is) immensely proud of him for graduating from high school and attending Linn Tech's automotive program for a year.

The fact was, then as now, that our nation had a need for more trade-school graduates who know and can apply practical trade skills. Dalton may one day be one of them. In the meantime, on more than one occasion, he helps Dr. Frick with her work at the clinic. As well, he has a following there made up of clients who like to book appointments when they know he is working the reception desk, because they enjoy his humor and conversations.

From the side, Rich Sandoval observed this stretch of Frick's life journey and was amazed at all she could accomplish on so many different levels. About her professional side alone, he concluded, "Ava was way beyond 'the boys.' She knew about medicines in Europe and the United Kingdom far beyond the understanding of most other doctors of her type here in the USA ... extremely impressive."

(If he only knew the other half of it!)

"Daisy, a happy, active Jack Russell Terrier (JRT), had parents who dressed her up in clothes or whatever matched the social occasion they were celebrating, be it Halloween, Thanksgiving, Christmas ... you get the idea.

"Now, a JRT (or a 'Terror-er' as I sometimes affectionately call them) is an outdoor, busy kind of breed, not precisely a girly-girl. And Daisy was a perfect example of this, one particular day, when she ran into the exam room, wearing a lacey-pink kind of dress. She sailed up onto the adjusting block and announced to me that she instead wanted to wear a baseball t-shirt ... and that it had to be one with blue pinstripes!

"I duly relayed that message to her parents. I hadn't made it up. I heard it clear as day, and was obliged to pass her message along."

* * *

About that time, a national TV network affiliate heard about Frick and what she could do. They sent a crew out to record an interview at her clinic. Later, airing the story, they dubbed her, "St. Louis' Animal Whisperer."

The thought alone of that brought and still brings a wry smile to Frick's face because it helped her help more animals, as would the next turn of the corner in her career.

In November 2015, Dr. Ava Lee Frick, awarded the prestigious honor of induction into the Animal Chiropractic Hall of Fame, was one of only four doctors selected to receive this distinguished recognition by a vote of her peers, certified chiropractors or veterinarians practicing internationally in the field of animal chiropractic. The selection was based primarily on contributions made to the development of the profession over 25 years.

* * *

CHAPTER 9: MIRACLE WORKER

By being and doing her best, Ava Frick attained a level of accomplishment and recognition among the "very best" of her profession. She also moved well beyond the status quo of many of her peers because of her charismatic approach to animals and their care, her uniquely intuitive ability to communicate with them, and a real give-and-take style that worked for her, which, oddly enough, had a quiet beginning.

"It was in 2003 when I had my first real definite 'whisper' moment. My son Dalton and I had gone to New Mexico to visit some friends, ride horses, and enjoy that terrain. The first evening in our friend's place, a dog from up the road, who had stopped by, was lying on the floor. I was setting the table, and Dalton asked my friend Jim what the dog's name was. Now, I was not even paying attention, but just as quickly as the question was posed, I instantly got a communication from the dog that his name was 'Dunkin.'

"Jim replied, 'We call him Bob. He just appeared in the neighborhood some time back.'

"I said, 'He said his name is Dunkin.'

"My friends did not seem willing to change what they called him, but Dunkin and I knew differently."

* * *

With regard to such abilities, Dr. Frick was not alone. She soon met a woman who also could easily understand such phenomena, Wendy Mettler-Wheeler.

Wendy was a sales-force manager and trainer extraordinaire married to a military colonel when she met Dr. Frick, whom she likes to call "Doc Ava," while she (Frick) conducted a seminar in 2001. After, they discussed the dogs that Mettler dearly loved. She had a special love for a dachshund she named "Yaeger" (after the famed experimental pilot) who lived with a debilitating physical problem: his auto-immune system was attacking his joints. Wheeler already had been to the University of Illinois Champaign campus, and there received a prescription for the drug Interferon to help reduce her dog's joint inflammation. The prognosis was not good for Yaeger's health to return, but Wheeler was not ready to throw in the towel on the canine's life. Other veterinarians she had visited delivered the same conventional "wisdom" to her: put Yaeger on Interferon and expect, at least, a better quality of life for his last year in existence. All had decided that Yaeger had only one more year to live, at best.

Fortunately, a female friend advised Wheeler to seek Doc Ava's guidance for supplements for Yeager.

Doc Ava considered Yaeger to be *"...an Alpha-male, a beautiful soul."* She told her new client, *"He's telling me he still wants to live."*

Together, on the spot, Doc Ava and Wheeler initiated a program designed to wean her boy off the pain killers now giving Yaeger stomach problems. Frick's prognosis was different than the others: *"Yaeger can have a far better life, and he can live for years to come."*

Yaeger did, in fact, recover his normal gait with Doc Ava's help and the coaching for daily handlings that she gave to Wheeler. He lived until 2013, seven or more years beyond the one year the other doctors had thought he would succumb.

Simultaneously, Wheeler had brought another of her favorite pets along for the ride because he hated being left at home. "Baron" was another dachshund with long red and tan hair.

"Baron was just walking around Doc Ava's clinic. He wasn't there for an appointment, but she noticed something about the way he was walking that didn't seem right. That day she took the time to examine him. Turned out, he was the one we thought was in good shape, but he needed help, too."

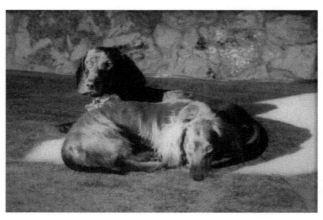

Baron & Yaeger

Baron, like his "brother" Yaeger, lived until he was 17, bringing Wheeler to recall, "Doc Ava and I worked in a partnership for those dogs. She is an animal communicator. She is the one there to help. Her attitude is one of 'How are *we* going to attack this?' and then we get to work on that plan."

But there was more!

Wheeler came across an older dachshund whose owner, an elderly woman, had died from cancer, leaving him alone, sitting in an open suitcase and waiting to travel. The family, not wanting the dog, took him to a pound in Chicago. The animal was 30 minutes away from euthanasia (because of his age and having contracted Kennel Cough).

Wheeler, by way of a rescue group, found out about his plight and decided to adopt him as a companion for her mother. His next stop was to Doc Ava's to get him started off right.

His name?

That came defiantly from the dog himself after Wheeler's Mom had suggested "Karl." Wheeler distinctly heard otherwise from him, sounding like a grumpy, old man, "No, not 'Karl!' … 'Copper'!"

Doc Ava was not the only one hearing outcries from aware animals. And Copper wasn't the last of the same kind of dog for which Wheeler sought her favorite veterinarian's guidance. Sometimes, it was for her friend's dogs, too.

"Princess Abigail" was a rescue dog, like Copper, and one of three dogs—two were males—let loose into a cornfield. Her foot pads were raw by the time someone found them. Living through that earned her a great home. Six years later, she was screaming with neck pain so severe their traditional veterinarian suggested either surgery or euthanasia. Wheeler had her own Alpha-Stim device and immediately initiated treatments the way she had done on her other dogs. After consulting with Doc Ava on what else to do, her report not long after that call revealed that Abigail was "spin-in-circles happy," according to Wheeler. The Princess lived another four years after her AST treatments.

>*"Our idea was to be pro-active, rather than reactive about whatever conditions were presented to us." –* Doc Ava

Wheeler explained, "Other vets preferred a no-relationship table manner, and Doc Ava actively and intentionally connects with the animals with a high-energy level, like with people, like human communication. [For pet owners], she educates about her philosophy, intending to make an impact. Yet, she knows when to back up, too.

"… With Baron, Doc Ava saw something and started him on a regimen that worked. With my mother-in-law's dog "Teddy," we sent hair samples to her, and her assessment was that a recent tooth cleaning showed positives for bacteria. Using her training and her perception ability, she found an organ in distress before worse conditions manifested. Doc Ava's caring is like going from Level One - mild interest (conventional vets) to Level Seven - care based on the idea of real help. Teddy, of course, responded well to what was recommended and to the way the Doc treated him."

For Wheeler, her "find" (Doc Ava) was so different, so much better, that she willingly made the 3.5-hour drive, each way, to see Dr. Frick every time one of her dogs needed help. The dogs sensed this difference, too. Once inside of her clinic, in Wheeler's words, "They act like jumping beans anxious for their turn to have Doc Ava talk to them and touch them, including the newest member of our clan, 'Zach.'"

Zach started out in an Illinois puppy mill. He was a piebald dachshund—they look a bit like a skunk. And, he was a survivor. His first owner never understood the repercussions of caging a dog for several years. Once let outside, he took off running into an area rife with desperate coyote packs, which, if forced to, could consider dog meat suitable nocturnal food. Scared from never having been let loose before, he ran for his life and hid from his owner. For days, 5:00 a.m. sightings were possible, but he remained too elusive for the search parties to pin him down and catch him.

Wheeler, too, had organized a search party, and they scoured local fields, storm drains, and gullies after most had given up the hunt, figuring Zach was dead. She remained vigilant until he, disoriented and shivering, trotted out of a cornfield. Spooked right away, he took off. Wheeler's husband ran in pursuit and attempted to snatch him up. Because it had been several days that the dog had food or protection from the elements, Lee was able to apprehend him before he ran back into the corn.

The most dramatic aspect of Zach's story was still to unfold: his next home was worse. The Illinois dachshund rescue group where he was taken placed him with someone they thought to be upstanding and qualified, but the woman turned out to be a hoarder. Investigators dressed in hazmat suits eventually entered the woman's basement and discovered it occupied by 54 cats, 40 of which were dead, nine other dogs, and Zach. Hearing of this, Wheeler determined that he would never suffer again. She was relentless in her fight to save him. Zach became her Number Three.

* * *

Dr. Frick's innate "Animal Whisperer" abilities were not as wild and "out there" as they appeared. And she was not an "only one." At times, the not-so-obvious communications she received from animals could be perceived by some of her animals' "parents."

Linda K. was first introduced to "Doc Ava" (She, too, liked to call Frick this way) a mere handful of years past the start of the 21st Century, when her family pup "Jake," a greyhound, developed issues with his spine. He wasn't able to use the stairs or jump in bed; he wasn't moving well at all. Linda and her family hurt just watching him struggle to get around. That's when her sister referred her to Dr. Frick's clinic:

"I was hesitant to drive the 50 miles from St. Louis to Union and back because I had young children. [The idea of] taking time in my busy day to drive to a doctor's appointment was foreign to me.

"After our first visit with Doc Ava, I realized the drive was no big deal, and we became regular clients. For Jake, Doc Ava prescribed supplements, Alpha-Stim, and chiropractic therapies. We went for it. Within a short amount of time, he improved and returned to his usual activities!

"Having become one of Doc Ava's biggest fans, I told everyone and anyone who ever mentioned an issue with their pets about the remedial work Doc Ava was able to do. Jake lived several more quality years under her care. We were, and are, incredibly grateful to 'my' Doc Ava."

Soon after, Linda's mom and dad, as well as her sister, also became regular clients at Doc Ava's clinic, drawn to her not only for her personal manner of caring but also because, as a doctor, she could think outside the box and heal or improve their pets' health issues as they age. The family members felt so strongly about the work she was doing, they began making donations in her honor to Frick's alma mater, University of Missouri College of Veterinary Medicine. Wanting the school to know how strongly they believed in Doc Ava's practice and quality of care, they spoke with school officials to see if they could establish a formal fund in her name. (A project still pursued.)

Linda adopted another greyhound, Cody, who developed diabetes at age eight. Because of his extraordinary care from Doc Ava, Cody lived to see 12 without losing his sight until the last few months of his life. Before he passed, he had endured many struggles associated with his diabetes: blood-sugar swings, weight loss, skin infections, cataracts, among other ills; yet, Dr. Frick was there every single step of the way, even making house calls when Cody was in severe distress and setting an excellent example for other pet owners as well as her peers.

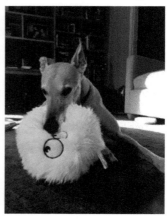
Cody

"Through Doc Ava's tweaks of Cody's supplement therapy, underwater-treadmill therapy, and the additions of whatever new she had studied, I learned to never give up hope. Her therapies brought Cody back from the brink of death, time, and time again … each time with an uncompromised quality of life. But, Cody, too, had a unique connection with Doc. I always was asking Doc Ava what she thought Cody was thinking—something I never would have asked of another veterinarian—once I saw that she has a special gift. She is an *extraordinary* veterinarian and person who, I believe, is a gift to treasure."

* * *

Maria Wakefield had earned her B.S. in Animal Science years earlier and then worked as a veterinarian nurse for 13 years, mostly with horses, by the time Standard Process hired her in 2011 as a Veterinarian Representative for Pennsylvania. During the time she studied the methodology and represented the products, as part of her approach to her position, she attended a Clinical Animal Nutrition Course that happened to have on the slate a seminar conducted by Dr. Frick.

Right away, she liked what she saw and heard from Frick. She enjoyed how she presented her data. Afterward, finding her to be approachable, Wakefield introduced herself.

"Dr. Frick was brilliant. She really knew her stuff! While other veterinarians were trained to approach their patients one way, there was something different about her. She reached outside the box, asking 'Why?' and other right questions. And the answers she had found gave people more options because she knew not only the traditional approach but also innovative ways to achieve better outcomes. And, she treated me like a person, answering all of my questions patiently."

The two hit it off as friends. To date, they have collaborated on two of Dr. Frick's books, including her *Hair Tissue Mineral Analysis Nutrition* publication.

"Dr. Frick is easy to work with. We collaborate over long-distance by phone calls and emails because she works with others like [they are] a person, not like a doctor, which instills confidence and trust in others like me. She sees, too, the benefit of working on projects on a gradient approach— never biting off more than we can chew at any one time, yet always advancing our work into a real [exchangeable] product."

* * *

Realizing anew that this world is still not a perfect one, not yet, Frick vowed to continue to help those who understood and cared for their animals—the one controllable area of her life where she could apply her skills and be acknowledged for the good that she produced. But, there were times when even the eternal optimist inside her wavered and pushed her to believe it may be time to give up. "Easy" was one of those times.

An 8-year-old, yellow Labrador, Easy had issues with his rear legs. Two MRI's showed pretty clear results: some arthritis in his left hip but otherwise no problems. His DNA had been checked for Degenerative Myelopathy, which came back negative. Doctors she had visited were unsure of what could be wrong, other than some other type of degenerative disease.

Having met him and performed her rudiments on him, Dr. Frick started Easy on supplements and AST. Still, he slowly, progressively worsened. In the summer of 2017, she started him on water-treadmill treatments, but, while he loved the water, the positive results that would enable him to function well at home were not forthcoming. By December, his back legs stopped working altogether.

Easy never exhibited pain; he seemed happy, and no one at Frick's clinic was ready to give up on him. Then (February 2018), his "parents" ordered doggie wheels for him and ... success! He loved them and began running all over the yard, playing with their other dog.

At this juncture, Dr. Frick suggested another round of AST. Having purchased the system in March 2018, her parents

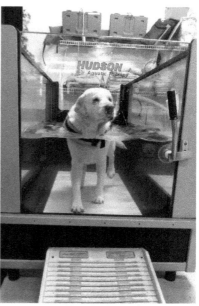

Easy in the underwater treadmill

commenced nightly 20-minute treatments. By the end of June, Easy started to stand up! Those involved with him were shocked, figuring this was just a fluke because he was standing on the concrete floor. Yet, he kept standing up … on grass, rugs, even a little on hardwood floors—something he had not done for at least a year!

Heartened, his owners let him slide down the ramp they had built for him to go outside … more success!

Easy continued to stand. Eventually, he could eat his breakfast and dinner this way. Though he clumsily walked himself outside to the grass, by now, he was walking without the doggie wheels and had not needed them for several weeks. By September, Easy had not used the wheels since June, and today, he walks and runs. He loves playing with the other dogs, and he walks up and down the stairs.

The continuous use of Alpha-Stim Therapy proved the winner. Easy's owners had thought he never would walk on his own, ever again. Now, they leash him because, otherwise, he chases after their neighbor's dogs!

"Without Dr. Frick, Easy would probably not be here— a stark contrast to other vets who had expressed little to no hope for him to live much longer. Because of her know-how, persistence, and communications with him, we are the lucky ones. We have Easy with us, happy and healthy again for what looks like many years to come," stated the owners.

Priceless.

And then there was "Gibson."

> *"A light Golden Retriever named*
> *Gibson comes for his initial visit. His*
> *'Mom,' Susan, brought him to see me*
> *because she was concerned that his*
> *behavior 'issues' might be pain-induced.*

"The next few minutes, I sit listening to what Susan is saying and describing from her perspective, noting that there is pity and a tone of sympathy in how she is relaying her story about him to me. Meanwhile, Gibson is lying near her by the bench she sits on ... his eyes visually distraught about something other than the fact that he has to be there.

"All of a sudden, he looks to me and tells me to tell her to 'STOP IT!' I mean, in no uncertain terms out of the blue, we have had a real cycle of communication: him to me, me getting it, and me to him, letting him know I get him.

"Then, without considering what I was about to say, I find myself speaking as his advocate, blurting out, 'He wants you to stop being that way with him. He hates it when you push sympathy on him. He doesn't like the way it makes him feel.'

"Susan, shocked, looks at me. We are each a little surprised.

"At that very moment, Gibson gets up, walks over to me— someone he had never seen before—and stands by me, slowly waggin' his tail and waitin' for me to pet him.

"I do, and just as quietly, he returns to sit beside his Mom. He's smiling, and the distraught look in his eyes is long gone.

*"Gibson's personality changed from
that day forward. He enjoys comin' to visit
and knows before they leave home where
he is going. From time to time, we've had
other conversations, always on his terms.
As things changed at home, his desire to
have me intercede on his behalf decreased.
But, I'm sure that he knows I am there for
him if he needs me."*

* * *

Want more? We are obliged:

Bunny, another Golden Retriever, had developed severe, chronic skin issues. Her owner exhausted the list of the best and brightest vets in her local area of San Diego County, California—a frustrating, expensive journey that left them both with no measurable results or changes in Bunny's condition.

Fortunately, Denise Rolen attended one of Dr. Frick's Alpha-Stim Training Seminars held at her clinic right about the time she was completely stumped about what to do regarding Bunny's health issues. Though Rolen was a holistic health practitioner for humans, she had no idea how to treat animals.

(Is that an indictment of the over-specialization trend in the healthcare fields for the past several decades? You be the judge.)

"Dr. Frick and I hit it off really well, and I kept in touch with her from California. She started treating Bunny by long-distance, using Fur Analysis. I had learned about Hair Analysis in my Metabolic Typing Advisor training and liked it. And now Ava told me about Analytical Research Labs (A.R.L.) in Phoenix, Arizona, where I proceeded to open an account and learn with her guidance all that I could about the process.

"When Ava offered her first Canine Nutrition classes, I signed up. Her wholly different approach started us on a regimen of home-cooked meals combined with *correct* supplementation based on the fur and bio-metric analyses.

"The result? Bunny lived without skin issues for the rest of her life, which turned out to be another seven years.

(R.I.P., Bunny. October 19, 2018.)"

* * *

In light cases and heavier ones, the consistent application of all of Dr. Frick's skills save not only many animals' health but also their lives. Case in point, "Ernest."

A stray, Ernest found himself in the clutches of an animal rescue center about to euthanize him when he got away somehow. The 12 to 14-year-old German Shepherd eventually passed out in a yard in North St. Louis, Missouri, discovered there by a passer-by who put in a call to Stray Rescue St. Louis. A dispatcher sent a truck to pick him up, though the caller had been unsure if the animal was dead or alive. Not much was expected at the site.

Ernest, however, was, indeed, alive! Barely so. The shelter took him in, where he languished in the pen assigned to him from his first day there. As the last straw, the staff texted a message about him to a 40-year-old woman they knew, named Julie. The team knew that she loved dogs, because she already had adopted at least 10 living at home with her.

Julie's dog-keeping philosophy was long-standing and straightforward:

"When I was a kid, I knew I was going to grow up and adopt old dogs. There was just something about them that captured my heart, so when I was old enough to have my own house, that's just what I did."

The caption under Ernest's image that the staff had sent to her was simple and to the point: "Hey, this looks like your kind of dog!"

Julie took him in, and that's how he came to be called "Ernest."

While trying to figure out the best way to care for him, for however long he had left to live—expectations were not high for long life, a friend told Julie about Dr. Frick, whom she said had helped her dog survive and even thrive after being severely bloated. Julie made an appointment with Dr. Frick.

Frick diagnosed Ernest's condition as showing horrible hip dysplasia (Hip dysplasia is a condition of weak hip sockets, which, over a lifetime, lead to severe arthritis or degenerative joint disease.) He had it really bad in his hips and elbows in combination with more arthritis that riddled his old body. She also informed Julie that since the tops of Ernest's ears were worn down and hairless, he probably had been an "outside dog" his entire life; and that his ear condition was the result of "flystrike." (The infestation of an animal by biting midges.)

Frick put Ernest on an assortment of supplements for his pain, arthritis, and the inflammation in his joints. She also recommended water therapy. Seeing her customer's confusion about the recommendation—*Ernest hobbles around as best he can,* was Julie's thought, Frick explained how the water would buoy his body weight and help loosen up Ernest's sore, arthritic elbows.

Julie's "lightbulb" went on, and she authorized the treatment enthusiastically.

Of course, Dr. Frick had been right about that! Ernest loved the water therapy even when he was just standing without walking. Gradually, he took a couple of steps in the tank.

That lesson and those to come later taught Julie a lot about her new veterinarian: "Just do what Ava says, because it always works … even when your mind tells you, 'Huh?'"

Stray Rescue St. Louis had estimated that Ernest was looking at only one to six weeks left to live when they adopted him out to Julie—a prognosis based on his body condition and severe heartworm infestation. However, with the supplements that Frick advised, Julie's care, and her patience, the water therapy and the AST treatments, Ernest pulled through his roughest times.

"32 weeks later, Ernest is still going strong!" exclaimed Julie.

Frick continued to see Ernest every few weeks to ensure that his menu of supplements was up to date with his changing condition, and for his ongoing chiropractic care.

As for Ernest's opinion of all this attention, Julie wrote in, "He just thinks he's going to visit the 'treats' people."

Truthfully, Ernest probably never had felt so good in his entire life! And Julie considers Dr. Frick, "Officially my not-so-secret weapon for all of my old babies!"

(NOTE: Ernest continued to flourish until he was bid farewell in June of 2019.)

* * *

At times, what Dr. Frick managed to do with her patients affected the well-being of the families who owned the animals. The following anecdote, one of many—this one from the Houser family, demonstrates how genuinely far-reaching her results have made a difference in other people's lives:

"In the Fall of 2011, I chatted with a burly guy holding a sweet little Dachshund in his ink-sleeved arms. He had taken her to a veterinarian in Union, Missouri, who miraculously had healed her back injuries and saved her life. He warned me, 'Be prepared, she's not going to be a typical veterinarian; she is going to do some things that will not be familiar to you, and you need to trust that it will work.'

"My older, sweet little Beagle-Dachshund mix, Pippi, was having intermittent neck and back issues, causing her debilitating pain and anxiety, and I had not been able to find her any relief. After the race, I looked up online, his doctor, Ava Frick, DVM.

"As I read about Dr. Frick, I thought about what he had said, but I was concerned that it would be expensive and not work, so I didn't do anything right away.

"Fast forward to April 2012. Pippi had another back and neck incident; this time, really serious. She had injured her neck and her upper back in a way that had her crouched and bent over in pain, hardly able to move. She screamed and cried every time she tried to walk or sit. She was defecating and urinating on herself and was unable to lay down. Also, she had stopped eating.

"Our veterinarian put her on a heavy dose of Rimadyl and Tramadol. After three days of no improvement and constant suffering, this doctor told me there was nothing else that could be done. "This may be the time to let her go," she said.

"As the last step, I called Dr. Frick's office, thinking *ultimately, if I have to euthanize Pippi, at least I will know I tried everything.* I explained that Pippi was in so much pain there was no possible way I could put her in the car and drive her 30-plus miles out to Union. The lovely woman on the phone said, "Not a problem. Take some Q-tips and swab the inside of her mouth; then, cut some fur from her tummy and bring it in."

"I left Pippi penned up in the kitchen, suffering and in pain, the day I visited Dr. Frick—a sad day for me.

"Arriving at Dr. Frick's office, I quickly understood this was going to be a different veterinary experience. Her clinic felt like a puppy spa. The consulting room was large, with lots of gym-like equipment. On a wall was an open cabinet filled with tiny vials.

"Dr. Frick and her assistant came into the room, and we had a brief introduction. I immediately shared a video of Pippi, crying as I showed her Pippi's condition and amount of pain. I asked her, 'Is there anything that can be done, or is it too late?'

"Dr. Frick replied nonchalantly, 'Of course, we can fix this. I've seen much worse.'

"Laying out the Q-tips and my little bit of Pippi's white fur on a bench, Dr. Frick pulled out boxes and opened bins containing jars of powders, liquids, and capsules. She brought out a long, narrow box that contained an instrument looking a lot like a conductor's baton. She then held the wand over the Q-tips, fur, and the little jars of pills and powders.

"Dispirited, I thought to myself, *Hmmm, what is going on here? Well, at least I know I have tried everything.* I asked Dr. Frick, 'So… how does this work?'

"'*Pointing at the bottles…*,' she replied, '*… It's like a cell phone: these are the numbers; the baton is the antenna, and I am that station.*'

"Hearing her explanation, I was a little hopeful.

"At the end of the 30-minute session, she handed me a small, brown paper bag full of supplements, homeopathic tinctures, and an electric-stimulation-therapy pack called Alpha-Stim.'

"On Dr. Frick's personal dog, Cheerio, her assistant showed me how to use the Alpha-Stim. (A patient and delightful Corgi, I might add.)

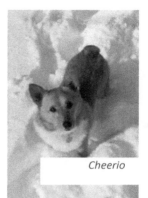

Cheerio

"Pippi was to receive four, 30-minute Alpha-Stim treatments per day, the supplements twice a day, and stop the Rimadyl.

"For the next four days, I followed the treatment plan exactly as instructed, using the supplements and Alpha-Stim therapy. By the fourth day, Pippi moved freely; she was eating and no longer crying in pain. By Day Seven, I was able to bring Pippi to see Dr. Frick for a follow-up appointment.

"It was simply amazing to watch how much better my sweet, little dog was doing in such a short amount of time. Dr. Frick went through the cycle with the baton again, adjusting and noting dosage changes for the powders, tinctures, and capsules. In the next 30 days, Pippi returned to her bright and sweet self—pain-free!

"Pippi remained on those supplements through the end of her life; she made it to 15 years. It was such a blessing to have her healthy those additional two-plus years, during which I started taking my older dog, Max, to Dr. Frick, who treated him for arthritis pain and dementia.

"We continue to take our current four-legged family to Dr. Frick. Our Pit Bull Terrier, Carmen, had a CCL injury (Cranial Cruciate Ligament, one of the most common injuries in dogs) a few years ago, and she was limping with serious, lack-of-mobility issues. Surgery was not a good option due to her older age and typical small bones and large muscle mass associated with her breed.

"Dr. Frick prescribed pain-management protocols that included anti-inflammation supplements and a 'toxic metals' assessment in her treatment plan. We were able to avoid any surgery.

"Today, Carmen is doing great; she's healthy and robust, and we couldn't be happier.

"Polly, our Lab/Pitbull mix and Mingus, our Siamese cat, also go to Dr. Frick for general wellbeing, joint care, and preventative/nutritional supplements.

"Dr. Frick always pinpoints the animal as her Number One priority. At times, she will be forthright to the guardian for not doing enough to support the well-being of the animal. Her commitment to animals is precisely why I respect her so much; why I have referred countless friends, and friends of friends to her veterinary practice. She is the most important doctor in our family. Her influence made visible to me the importance of alternative healthcare not only for my animals but also for my husband and me. I continue to learn from her about the values of functional medicine, supplementation, joint care, inflammation reduction, quality nutrition, and bodily toxins removal. Every time visiting, I learn something new about good health, which benefits my entire family and me.

"We are so grateful for our Dr. Frick, who has been a true guardian and guide for good health. Beyond words."
— Sue Harken-Houser & Chip Houser; Carmen, Mingus, and Polly (in loving memory of Max and Pippi).

A lovely testimonial.

* * *

"Our horses are specially selected and trained for their career at Ride-On St. Louis, a nonprofit therapeutic horsemanship program. They are our partners, conditioned athletes, and working service horses with a clearly defined job, training, and exercise routine. Dr. Frick is key to making this a reality, and she has been a great support to the care and health we must give our equine team. Because of her attention to detail and ability to see subtle changes in their posture and function, we are able to reduce the downtime and keep them in the program for many years beyond the traditional. We pride ourselves on producing and maintaining happy, healthy, willing horses who enjoy their role, and provide them with the highest quality care and conditioning so they may thrive in their own personal lives and produce the best outcomes for our clients." — Marita Wassman, Director & Founder Ride-On St. Louis.

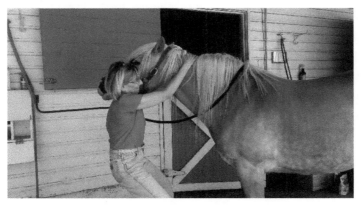

Dr. Ava gives April a cervical adjustment

***

Trenna Edwards-Quevreaux' story of two of her kitties tells another angle of Dr. Frick's story well:

My husband and I first heard about Dr. Frick on a camping trip, when a mutual friend brought someone along who had taken her pets to Dr. Frick for several years. She mentioned that Dr. Frick's approach was "very different" than any other veterinarian she had ever met but was also amazed at her success with healing her rescue dog back to health for an additional three years, when every other vet was recommending euthanizing, all while using those dreaded words of "it's time." This is every pet owner's nightmare, as we had just gone through this several months earlier, and we weren't so lucky.

Hearing our new friend's story piqued our interest a great deal as we follow a very natural and holistic approach ourselves, and treating our animals in the same way just made perfect sense to us. When we got home, we immediately made an appointment with her. We saw near immediate improvements in mobility with our very senior Maine Coon and witnessed him being able to jump up to the bathroom sink again, after just a few weeks of treatment. WOW! This was truly remarkable as he seemed to have reasonably significant arthritis, and to see him make such an improvement was quite a noteworthy occurrence.

The most miraculous event, though, was yet to come. My husband and I went out of town over a long weekend, and when we returned, we noticed that our nine-year-old Persian kitty, Esther, was refusing to eat, which was very odd as she was always a very voracious eater. By the next morning, her condition had deteriorated rapidly. Dr. Frick was out of town, so we rushed her to a cat clinic close to our house to see what the problem was. It was some of the worst news we could have imagined, she was in acute liver failure, per the blood work. The veterinarian's prognosis was profoundly grim. In shock, we rushed her to a specialty clinic and were told that she had a condition called cholangial-hepatitis, and would need a feeding tube. We were sent home with a lot of medicine, feeding tube care and instructions, and were told she should start to feel better and eat on her own in a few days. She was hospitalized three more times in the next two weeks, and had continued to decline even further – her liver enzymes were even worse than they were initially. The guesswork of changing her medicines was frustrating, and after all of this, there was still no attempt to eat. Now the blood work was showing that she was also in kidney failure.

After a month, there was still zero improvements, and we were finally able to take her to Dr. Frick. As I had strongly suspected, none of the medicines the specialty clinic was giving her were what her little body needed to heal. Our amazing Dr. Frick worked with her, and within a day and a half, she was eating on her own. Within one week, she no longer required tube feedings. Within roughly one month, the blood work demonstrated what I felt had happened; her liver and kidney failure were reversed entirely. She had even gained her weight back and was able to get her feeding tube removed.

My story is not to disparage traditional veterinarians, as I have tremendous gratitude for the specialty clinic for the feeding tube, because, without it, she surely would have died. However, if we hadn't taken her to Dr. Frick for treatment, which was completely different than all treatments recommended to us by standard western veterinary medicine, I am sure she would not be with us today. The type of practice that Dr. Frick has is genuinely miraculous for so many pets and their owners, and each day we are so, so thankful for that fateful camping trip.

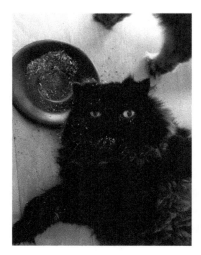

Esther's in catnip heaven!

* * *

In 2016, not one to rest on her laurels, Dr. Frick developed and presented to the world at a conference her *Tai Chi-huahua* low-impact exercise program for animals. At her fully operational clinic in Eureka, Missouri, now named Pet Rehab & Pain Clinic, more books, articles, and DVDs are part of her menu of products designed to be helpful for her peers and the lay public.

However, her recognition, awards, and forward progress failed to bring closure to an ongoing problem she faces:

> *"... how to convince people that I*
> *really know what I know? That I can,*
> *indeed, 'see' beyond the obvious?"*

Looking at an animal, Dr. Frick sees in their posture or gait what most others do not. If something non-optimum is occurring, she sees that and what the condition does to their other body parts, not because she is odd or unusual but because she takes "*... more responsibility for the life and condition of the animal in her sights.*"

Evidence of her responsibility level exists in her vicinity: rarely have general practitioner veterinarians, outside of university professors, had an acclaimed book published by an international publisher. Few have also written and seen their articles or white papers published four times in leading veterinarian journals and in a scientific research journal. She has represented two major, industry-related nutritional and treatment companies while maintaining an ongoing practice utilizing veterinary medicine, animal chiropractic, and other modalities. She lectures across America, has established worldwide nutritional courses for students of the science and established herself as a bonafide pioneer in animal rehabilitation.

Why? Because, while dodging arrows from others within her industry with tenacity, she stayed focused on her purpose and vision *for the animals.* In other words, she held her ground and stayed the course of her core responsibility.

Dr. Frick is in a race—a hot pursuit of new and innovative solutions because of not wanting one single animal to be euthanized needlessly, to suffer for one more horrific minute, or to, abandoned, die unnecessarily, when correctly applied rehabilitation can recover so much life.

Dr. Frick finds unique ways to offer desperate people— the animal owners who come to her—renewed hope and reassurance. When others believe nothing can be done about it, she believes that something CAN, more often than not, be done about an ill or injured animal.

Pivotal incidents in her life enhanced her ability to observe, to know what she sees, and to speak out about what she finds so that others, hopefully, take a closer look, see what is there to see, and not cling to the status quo of what "should or should not be done."

Dr. Frick, an expert in chiropractic, whole-food nutrition, microcurrent therapy, exercise physiotherapy, and hair tissue mineral analysis, is restless. She is not a hoarder of her knowledge—a good thing:

> *"Not one to believe everything taught*
> *me was gospel, my conviction remains to*
> *seek and learn more, accepting*
> *responsibility for the knowledge that I*
> *study and own and transferring my*
> *confidence to each animal owner willing to*
> *believe in me and what I know to be true."*

* * *

In today's Millennial vernacular, Frick has been *"crushing it"* for decades by looking, seeing and studying, and informing her peers of her findings as well as educating and edifying her clients and their animals to be self-reliant.

One would think that would be enough; that the gods of Karma would be satisfied by her work; but, we live in a dangerous environment here on Earth. Sometime around 2018, something happened to Frick's stamina. The changes made her ability to push her purpose and do her work even more challenging. Accustomed to informing a client that their pet has a disease condition, she fell ill to one of her own: a diagnosis of Lyme Disease followed an examination of her individual complaints of symptoms. Her reply to the news was to simply start learning more about Lyme.

> *"I am dealing with 'creatures' within*
> *my body. Needing more facts and answers,*
> *yet not wanting to fuel my enemy, I began*
> *a new adventure. Parallel to my treatments*
> *with dogs—I deal with their ups and downs*
> *and mood changes all the time—I now*
> *treat my own!"*

From the accumulated unpleasant events in her life—Lyme is one of them—Dr. Frick gleaned a step-by-step formula for decision-making, which she applies to herself religiously:

1. Take responsibility for what has happened.

2. Assess the situation and discover what caused it in order to avoid getting into a similar situation.

3. Find a solution or a way to deal with it, and, for Frick, ask, "What do I now do to help (two- and four-legged) others?"

> *"My formula moves me away from 'dis-ability' to 'respons-ability,' enabling me to respond quickly and effectively to change the wrong course for the better. I am tackling the Lyme and making Lyme-ade for myself and others!"*

Applying her formula, she continued to work and bring help to her clients, including one Nancy Radtke, "Dr. Frick helped my 'boy,' Max, when everyone else had given up on him."

In July of 2018, Max developed bloat—Gastric dilatation and volvulus syndrome (GDV), more commonly referred to as gastric torsion or bloat in dogs. Their stomach dilates and then rotates, or twists, around its short axis. He needed emergency surgery. Pre-op blood work revealed his kidney values already weakened dangerously.

The ER Vet told Radtke that she was afraid the anesthesia would "fry" Max's kidneys and, as a result, he wouldn't live long following the surgery. She recommended that Max be euthanized and left the decision to Radtke, who opted to move forward with the surgery.

Following his surgery, Max struggled to get better. On the third day after, a dire prognosis came. A subsequent follow-up visit to his traditional veterinarian was not encouraging, either. His life expectancy was two weeks, at best.

Radtke decided to consult Dr. Frick, and she scheduled an appointment:

"I will be forever grateful that I made that decision," Radtke remembered "… My 'boy' continued to improve and thrive and his visits were especially encouraging. Dr. Frick was thrilled with his progress and his response to the therapy and medications that he received from her."

Almost eighteen months out (as of late 2019) from his expected "last days," amazed and thankful cannot describe the way her family feels about his turn for the better.

"All thanks to Dr. Ava Frick, to her faith, knowledge, and treatment of Max."

* * *

CHAPTER 10: VIRTUES & COMMUNICATION

People visit Dr. Frick mostly out of concern for the conditions of their pet animals than about her accumulated experience, accredited diplomas, awards, and recognitions. Still, she is a real, live, spiritual human being (like the rest of us)—one who gathers her strengths from several sources, including her environment. She is often inspired by, in her words,

> *"... the sound of drums in a marching band, the beat of a really great two-steppin' song, or an Indian flute wafting across an open-desert canyon...*

> *"Some days it's... the smell of fresh-cut hay, leather, a spring rain, the inside of a barn, a one-month-old kitten, or bacon cooking on the stove...*

> *"Yet, other moments ... the sight of the Grand Canyon, fall colors of leaves on trees, white caps on a rolling river, or a solid-hit baseball ... that takes me to another dimension...*

> *"The feel of water gently rocking my canoe back and forth, of rising out of the*

water on skis pulled by a boat, of smooth,
shiny stones, or a cantering horse between
my legs ... the rumble of a motor's sound
exiting a large tailpipe, and how my chest
reverberates its cadence.

"All of it reminds me that I am
experiencing life, that I am alive!

"... And from that, I take inspiration,
as well as from people doing kind deeds
for one another, the smiles on the faces of
little children, or the ability of one man
who builds an entire house ... and heroes."

* * *

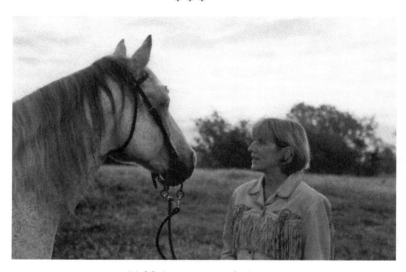

Mel & Ava... contemplating...

Whatever her motivations and inspirations as a person, a veterinary doctor, and animal chiropractor, the common denominator among Ava Frick's relationships to her family, her staff, her patients, and their owners are *communication.*

In fact, communication is the avenue on which is built all understanding. There are so many ways to accomplish a real connection… and a few that will not.

> *" I do remember one time a couple of parents looking at their older, sick pet and thinking it was just too much trouble for them to keep.*

> *"I knew the pet could be helped, but they wanted me to tell their kids it was too sick and needed to be euthanized for its welfare.*

> *"Of course, you know my answer: I told them I absolutely would not agree to any such discussion as that was not my belief."*

The outcome of that exchange was lost in the shuffle of ideas; in other words, the animal's needs disappeared on the parents' unwillingness to listen and heed a trained veterinarian doctor's advice. What *seemed like* communication was merely verbiage and inaction based on the couple's fixed, perverted idea of what help should be.

> *"Some people at that point will go into a tirade of how a veterinarian is supposed to 'help' animals ... like it is our obligation to take on their responsibility just to make their life easier.*

> *"I have been actually hollered at over refusing a nonsensical PTS (put to sleep)."*

In actuality, real communication is simple to learn and to apply, once the definitive formula for its composition is grasped.

Excellent communication inevitably brings about understanding, which, in turn, enhances outcomes, predicts behavior, and determines courses of action.

Dr. Frick's anecdotal stories about animals in this book and the outcomes she has effected upon different animals are living proof that real communication is not only possible but also leads to higher survival potential and longer lives, both animal and human.

Also, there is the matter of QUALITY of communication. To communicate is an ability. Like other abilities, one must practice to make it better and more natural. Veterinarians wanting to go outside of the box from what they were furnished in vet school, and people owning pets and caring about them beyond normal, must learn more about the connection of communication to understanding and practice it. Dr. Frick has applied such data for years, which has contributed to her recognitions and, more importantly, her results with animals.

And, after all, that is the point, isn't it?

We live on this whirling ball of a planet—humans, and animals together—to enhance or worsen relations among ourselves. Our survival and the quality of our races depend on our understandings of each other.

For Dr. Frick and her peer veterinarians and animal chiropractors, the common-denominator factor of interest is help—how to help the symbioses of animals and humans. Their work is of paramount importance—what we do or fail to do will affect the lifespans of our races for good or bad. Quite factually, we NEED each other; we can and should give and take from each other. We MUST learn to understand how to care for each other better because our very existence depends on how much *real* inter-species communication we can and do employ.

And, perhaps, that is the most important lesson and legacy of Dr. Frick's lifetime.

Dr. Frick is a leading proponent of this philosophy. She is a beacon, a lighthouse, which shows us the way past the shoals to clean, open waters.

Seeing what she sees is possible for the rest of us. Believing that she knows what she knows is also possible. Proof will come when more animal doctors and animal owners take on the same responsibilities that Dr. Frick already takes *to look and to listen to what animals tell us all the time.*

Personal frustration about what an animal does or doesn't do escalates emotions of unkindness and turmoil and depresses survival potential. Frustration turned to anger, beatings, kicking, and widespread animal abuse are evidence of someone's inability to communicate, and not just with animals.

The inability to confront (be there) and communicate brings war. Yet, war is unnecessary between animals and people. Animals communicate the ways they know how. They do what their instincts tell them to do for one common reason only: survival.

An animal's focus attunes solely to its survival, whereas Man's outlook can be more than that. Man has his reason, intelligence, and spirituality. He has a full panoply of choices. Therefore, a lack of real communication—human to animal—is not their fault but a *human* fault and a failure to understand their needs or wants.

Humans, being sentient spiritual beings (for the most part), should understand and act better than to take out their frustrations on animals and abuse them.

"I have found it funny when a dog and
cat in a home are interacting, one trying to

*get the other to stop, each using
vocabulary and body lingo specific to their
species: the puffed-up cat ... back arched,
tail widened, eyes like saucers, raised on
tippy toes...*

*"... The dog with ears laid back, nose
and lips curled, teeth exposed, and
snarling...*

*"... Both species doing their best to
tell the other to stop and get lost, and
neither with the vaguest notion their
message will not cross the divide.*

*"Dog-to-dog, they would have gotten
the message. Cat-to-cat, they would back
off, or mount the attack...*

*"... But, in cross-species
conversation, both sides are surprised
when their best attempts to communicate
fall on deaf ears annoyingly, no doubt."*

* * *

We learn from Dr. Frick's astute observations that understanding is the most significant result of real communication between our species and the animal world; yet, for that outcome three other factors need to be in place:

1. The will to face up to whatever it takes to communicate about and to resolve a problem;

2. The interest to care enough about another or other parties;

3. Shared agreement or, at least, a mutual reaching out for agreed-upon reality with another or

others about what is being discussed and/or handled.

Assuming those three points are in place, a flow of granting beingness (letting them be who they are) toward an animal is crucial. Dr. Frick literally tells them they are fantastic, pretty, or handsome; that they move well, or have lovely eyes; at times, she might just thank them for being there to begin sharing the same space together, accenting the positive.

"In the old days, before we knew how harmful it was, when a thermometer broke, and its mercury spilled onto the floor in small beads, we could move them and watch them instantly coalesce into a larger droplet. The transition happened instantaneously. And so it goes with animals I come into contact with."

* * *

We know from Dr. Frick's early experiences with barn cats and, later, with one large, rabid dog that the outcomes of attempts to communicate are not always predictable. She learned early that not all animals liked her. After many years, however, she "tuned in" by training for Animal Chiropractic certification. Chiropractic taught her specific gentle-motion palpation skills, to which she never had been exposed in the field of veterinary medicine. Using less pressure and smaller movements, she learned to "read" more with the tips of her fingers than perform indiscriminate joint or spinal examinations the way her vet school training dictated. In her words, *"...[That was] such an eye-opener!"*

There were larger animals she cared about and wanted to help, too. (The bigger the heart, the more significant the caring.)

"Because horses were a pleasure for me, I never wanted to have them as part of my veterinary practice. I also didn't want my horses to be the ones left out. You know, 'the cobbler's kids don't have shoes' deal?

"When chiropractic came along ... different story, because I was not doing anything painful to them. I was making them feel better. Horses are very 'in tune' and 'into' their bodies. They tell you when it feels good, and they let you know when it doesn't."

* * *

The typical curiosa that Dr. Frick faces is: "It must be difficult knowing what to do since they can't talk to you." Her reply is that they talk to her all the time.

Animals communicate much more than most humans observe.

"My job as a communicator to animals is to discover what they feel or think (their reality), observe how much effort they are using to make sure I get the point, check back in with them that what I am about to do is correct for their need for comfort, do what is needed, and let them have the moment of relief.

Some buck up into the adjustment, like saying, 'Come on, do that! Let's get 'er done!' And they always make me laugh when they do that.

*"Often, they will just turn and look
straight at me, as if to say, 'Thank you.'
And then I am their newest best friend,
which makes it all worthwhile."*

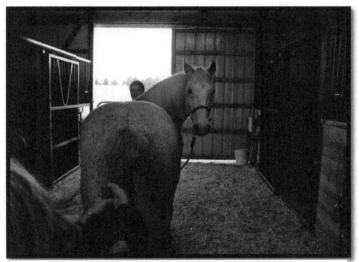

Tail traction on one of the horses

* * *

No doubt, for both doctor and animal.

Dr. Frick's ability to give and receive communications from animals extended across other species, including, believe it or not, birds. Simply put, as her life and career progressed, she learned different ways to communicate not only with people but also several other species.

Birds—many people know this, especially parrots, are capable of a unique perception of human, even animal, conversation, and word application. In their peculiar, guttural way, they can mimic the ring of a phone, meows of cats, and the exact tone of a person's voice at home. Some learn many words, though apparently unaware of their meanings.

Take a look at Sailor the McCaw, who, lacking attention for some time and being isolated, had taken to feather plucking. Now a hideous looking bird, he was starved for attention and was still trying to communicate, even though his word selection was sub-optimal:

"My first close encounter with a talking bird was a McCaw named 'Sailor.' He had been offered up to the College of Veterinary Medicine Small Animal Clinic for being a feather picker.

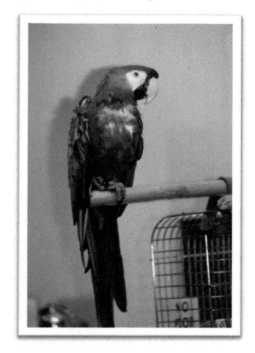

Salty Sailor

"Feather picking commences when these highly social birds become extremely upset or stressed, and they have no way to resolve the situation. It appears, then, that they feel helpless. Well, it was Dr. Renniger, a resident, who had taken Sailor 'under his wing' in an effort to help him.

"The busiest and most pleasant place was the small animal Intensive Care Unit (ICU), and there is where he hung out.

"The students on that rotation took shifts twenty-four/seven. One of my classmates, forever known to us as 'RG' and whose real name shall be withheld, was fluent with four-letter words. They flowed out of his mouth without a blink of his eye like hot wax spilled on a car hood in summer. And when RG worked the late night/early morning shift, he liked to talk to himself, as well as to Sailor, words that Sailor decided on his own to learn and mimic.

"One day Dr. Cynthia Trimm, the Board Certified Anesthesiologist at the clinic, was touring a group of visiting veterinarians and educators from Japan. Impressed with his audience of foreigners, Sailor showed off, delivering a barrage of his newest vocabulary additions.

"The more Dr. Trimm tried to ignore him and make little of his presence, the louder and louder Sailor screamed out his menacing trail of four-lettered words!

*"Needless to say, Sailor was moved
under duress to a different location… way
off campus."*

* * *

Birds are receptive to other perceptions in their vicinity and, not knowing the significance for humans of their messages, they are willing to talk. In this regard, Lanie Frick's bird story seemed appropriate to re-state here, and in her words:

"While away on a trip, I scheduled my parents to go over and feed animals for me. One of my compadres at the time was a double-yellow-headed Amazon parrot I had named 'José.' I left him safely secured in his large cage located in my studio, which included a bathroom, a freezer, and a storage area.

"On one of the feeding trips, my sister Ava was at the house visiting, so she went with my parents on the feed chore.

"When they walked into the studio, Jose' started raisin' a ruckus like he was trying to tell them something. Then they caught a whiff of his upset state: a BIG STINK was permeatin' the room!

"But, they thought, *what is he trying to say?* That's when Ava deciphered his bird lingo, 'The toilet! The toilet!' which he kept repeatin.' So, they checked the toilet, but that was fine.

"Then, Dad thought about the freezer. Yep, that was it. The circuit breaker had gotten tripped, and everything in the fridge was beyond thawed out!

"Jose' didn't have the concept of what a freezer was, but he knew a stink when he smelt one, and he wanted it taken care of and gone. And that's precisely what they proceeded to do, making José once again a happy bird."

"After all, José had the intent to get the message across that the odor was not him! And we heard what he was telling us."

Not to be outdone by her sibling Lanie, Ava recalled a bird story of her own, involving her clinic and its staff.

"Some time ago, a bird came to visit us at my Animal Fitness Center east of Union.

"Joan, an employee, had gone outside to clean up the front. She quickly came back inside, surprised that there was a small parrot in the big elm tree near the entrance, so we all headed outside to see this bird. When we got there, the bird decides to 'come on down,' and it landed on Joan's shoulder.

"It was apparent this is a distressed bird, for it had very few feathers. The body is pitifully bald. It sat there as we went inside.

"Where did she come from? we all thought. A guess was from the new apartment buildings getting filled on the east side of the property.

"She must have had a terrible life, and could have totally been set 'free' in an effort to get rid of her and reduce their conscious struggle for lack of caring for her was my thought. She has found her

way to a place of peace and love. Now, what to do?

"I had two exam rooms. One was to be denoted the bird space, for now.

"Dalton had some old hamster cages that we took apart and rigged up like perches. Next, we went to Wal-Mart (less than a mile away) and got some emergency bird food for the evening. Then we began an internet search for how to help her more.

"Each morning, I would get there early and take care of her space, water, food, as well as carry on conversations. In return, she looked on in silence. Over the next few days, she began to mimic my client conversations. She could be heard through the wall vent grate, muttering a spattering of words as if answering in reply to questions. None at this point distinct.

"Later in the week, on my morning visit, I talked to her and tried to get her to climb up on my arm and shoulder. Looking at her, while I'm using sentences to encourage her to take the next leap of trust, she straightens up her back just a bit, raises her head, looks right at me, and says, 'Step up?'

"I am ecstatic ... a breakthrough! She speaks to me!

"Is that your word? I say. 'Step up?
Go ahead, yes, step up.'

"And that is precisely what she did.
Reaching out one leg, then withdrawing
quickly as if in hesitation that I am not
where she wants to go, she takes the first
step. Gripping on, she sidesteps all the
way up my arm.

"At that point, I think we were both
smiling with satisfaction."

* * *

Within a month, a client, who had a parrot just like her, came, thrilled to have found a mate. The original house bird eventually regrew all her feathers, showing everyone that life was good, and she was happy.

Dr. Frick slept well that night. Her customers and staff did, too. Good living follows her, just like the Pied Piper.

* * *

CHAPTER 11: THE CYCLE OF HAY

Many people may never realize the time, efforts, and man/woman power that caring for one or more horses consumes. You have to have owned one to know.

"As Moe, a good friend of mine from Arizona related about a less than an agreeable buddy, whose wife had gotten him a horse, 'Horses eat money and poop work!'"

* * *

Take hay, for instance: once grown, and the June/July Missouri weather cooperates, hooking up the mower to a tractor is the thing to do to get it cut and square-baled—actually a rectangle but called square-baled to compare against large, round bales.

Next, a farmhand pitches up the bales from the ground onto a flatbed trailer pulled by a tractor and its driver, as another workhand stacks them in alternating patterns, so they are tight and stay put. The fully loaded wagon is driven to an elevator lift positioned at ground level under a side-opening leading to a barn loft. The bailer then tosses bales onto the elevator, and another receives and stacks them in the barn loft.

From there, if only feeding their livestock, farmers get the hay tossed down as needed and shared with the horses—non-farmers make a purchase, after which those bales are restacked onto a truck bed in a tight, alternating pattern and hauled to the owner's barn and re-stored there.

Actual feeding requires the bales to be cut open and flaked out to the horse(s) in their stalls. Once consumed, the cycle begins anew.

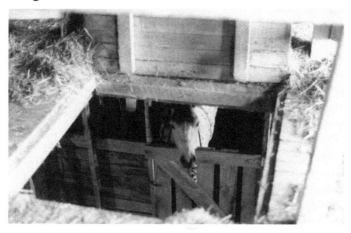

Waiting for the hay to fall...

Leftover hay, called "manure," gets pitchforked into a wheel barrel. Once all stalls are picked, the wheel barrel is pushed out to a manure mound that accumulates until the pile is large enough to be removed, again bringing into play the tractor to haul the manure remnants to a field for use as fertilizer—a cycle of tasks similarly done on trail rides, when horse riders camp out for

Lanie wields another wheelbarrow load of barn manure.

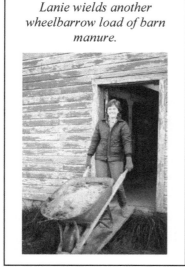

several days. On the farm, the rule is: wash, rinse, repeat, and repeat over and over again—another factor of life and living.

In farm living, some people are cutters, some compressors, and some tossers, stackers, pickers, consumers, or haulers. From birth, we get taken care of by others, toted here and there, and plopped down in strange places. Most people we meet along our ways help us find our "It"—what motivates us. Seeing this "It" adds proper fuel to our efforts to achieve our goals. Finding this purpose, we get it applied. In the end, once again, we get hauled by others here and there.

Fortunately, recycling happens. We get "do-overs" because of who we *really are*, immortals all.

Wanting to make an impact on others and to improve our lives and theirs, we wonder: *What am I made of? Do I, like hay, offer high-quality, nutritive ingredients to the game and its players? Am I tasty? Nourishing? Good enough to help others live their lives better?*

> *"I sure hope so, for that is why I'm*
> *here on Earth this go-round: to help others*
> *be better. Because of my upbringing, my*
> *professional choices, and my, at times,*
> *easy-to-take and painfully hard-to-swallow*
> *heritage, I will never again look at hay and*
> *manure piles the same way."*

* * *

There is love, and there is unconditional love. This is the "why" behind so many people caring for animals. No matter what the situation, an animal's love is never about *things*; it is solely about YOU.

Pure, no-strings-attached love is why people will go to great lengths to save the animals they love; the animals *always* love them back.

> *"Dogs like us; they like to be around people. Cats, on the other hand, like naps. And horses love to run free. All of these animals share a love for food, albeit dogs will mostly eat what you give them; cats will eat only by their choice, and horses, like fishes, will eat and eat until they kill themselves ... so you have to treat each one for who they are."*

* * *

CHAPTER 12: THE POT O' GOLD

While her Dad Dennis and her Grandpa Owen were not religious—a Frick family trait dating back to the 1800s in Germany—both were 32nd-degree Masons of the Scottish Rite, an organization that places God, ethics, and morals at the forefront of their lives. Ava's Mom Sarah was a member of the Eastern Star. The younger Ava reflected both her parents' leanings by becoming a Rainbow Girl, their only daughter to do so.

The International Order of Rainbow for Girls (IORG) is an organization for young women aged 11 to 20, which teaches training through community service. Founded in McAlester, Oklahoma in 1922, the Rainbow Girls believes that each color of the rainbow (red, orange, yellow, green, blue, indigo, and violet) represents a path of life. Similar to the Masonic Lodge, the IORG's goal is to instill decision making based on God. Following their purpose, it helps young girls make better choices in life guided by faith, hope, and charity. As such, it made a difference in Ava's experience as a young girl and, later, as a woman.

Once Ava turned the corner at 40 and again asked why, she began to create more ideas of expansion. With each big brainstorm, she got excited, thinking *maybe this one is my pot o' gold! Now I will be wealthy!*

With each new notion ... the spinal laser pads, the canine, and feline Clinical Animal Nutrition Survey, finding Alpha-Stim Therapy, developing equine exercises into a published book, and moving her clinic closer to St. Louis … Ava's mind would get going to where at night she would pray to God, asking him to please turn it off.

"I was anxious to get to the pot o'
gold and seize the monetary reward, but
my rainbow wasn't done being painted.
Time—the accumulation of wins and
losses—like a rainbow was quickly fading
in the sky. To appreciate that there needed
to be a gathering, took aging. Early on, the
pot was not full (to me), and the rainbow
dim.

"I realized, recently, that none of
those events and ventures was meant to be
the pot o' gold. Each was, instead, only
one band of color in my rainbow. The red,
orange, yellow, green, blue, indigo, and
violet … when all of those bands are
completed, there the gilded pot will be.

"I have thought the 'Pot O' Gold'
brought money, but that's not it at all.
Instead, it is my collection of contributions
made to society. Also, my reward; a
reward measured in pleasures: raising a
good son, jobs well done,
accomplishments, fulfilling my purpose for
being here at this point in time, completing
the bucket list, helping others, contributing
to saving the planet, doing what I believed
was right, keeping my conscience (my
integrity) and guarding my ethics (sense of
good reason toward survival for all).

*"Yes, my pot o' gold is about more
than money; yet, there's gotta be some
extra cash at the bottom of that pot!*

*"Like a Leprechaun, I am lucky that I
always have known, generally, my
purpose. I just tweaked it a bit over the
years."*

* * *

For others, finding purpose may be harder because it may be hidden. They will have to work to dig it out from under false purposes. Still, with work and faith, the winning may be more significant and the self-satisfaction deeper.

*"I believe God, the Supreme Being,
gives us permission to be all things good.
And, though life can seem so twisted, at
times, that remains a part of everyone's
purpose for being here."*

* * *

Those who enjoy and appreciate sharing Earth with animals know that a part of our responsibility is to learn from them; to be alert and aware about their styles of communication, not only for each species but also for the individuals within them; and to acknowledge their communications and accept their inevitable invitations to dance.

Animals teach us to love unconditionally, to laugh, to have compassion, to be patient, and, at times, to listen to the quiet. They show us the values and virtues of affinity, agreement, understanding, responsibility, cautiousness, and how to think, share, admire, and survive. Through animals, we can decipher not only empowerment but also forgiveness. And, that not everyone likes us but somehow that is okay.

Animals share with us their companionship, how to be warriors, and how to die.

Conversely, Ava Frick's life story here is what is not only her truth but ours, because we, along with her, *can* know the realities of animals.

Animals and humans sharing Earth are like dancing in so many ways. Doing chiropractic, physiotherapy, and other exercises with animals are Ava Frick's responses to that dance: how she asks for the partner's permission to co-exist, grants beingness and self-importance temporarily, accepts their invitations, and validates their (good or bad) feelings and expressions of concern.

We are the better for her life because from her we can learn what to do when and how an invitation to dance is being extended to us.

Accepting the invitation teaches us that we can be kind and helpful; that, in the end, we always can thank our partner for the dance, no matter how it turned out because we get our "do-overs" (lifetimes) as Ava calls them.

If the animal world has an "It" and its related choices, species by species, so, too, must Humanity have its "It." Humans—we are spiritual beings having human-body existences—will continue to play mind-games on themselves and each other; yet, by allowing animals the right to their games the same way we have a similar right to ours, whether the same, similar, or different, we will all survive better. We will all flourish and prosper.

"For me, my 'It'—what leads my way—is animals."

Well, you're here on Earth. Find your own, "It."

* * *

CHAPTER 13: LOOKIN' AHEAD

In 2017, Dr. Frick took more steps into the future of animal healthcare modalities by continuing her research of innovative Herbal Phytotherapy—*"Herbs are nature's drugs"*—applications, including the positive and negative effects of herbs versus drugs. This motivated her budding interest in understanding Ayurvedic medicines and the three doshas (Dosha, the energy that defines body makeups) - Vata, Pitta, and Kapha - relative to animals.

As always, her aim was to enable animal bodies to heal, using a natural extension of the long histories developed in India of using herbs from that region of the planet.

A pet owner named John, who loved his Bernese Mountain Dog Bernie, became one of her first test subjects for her new nutritional-balancing approach. The dog had fallen off a bed and hurt himself. John took him for an MRI, but in the process of Bernie getting prepped, a thoracic mass was discovered near the heart. The MRI was canceled. John returned to Dr. Frick for therapy and more help since Bernie's diagnosis and long-term life expectancy were not good.

John had a friend, Michelle, who had been married to a Hindi, with whom she practiced Ayurveda. She was to be in town soon, and John requested her help to find a diet that would fit Bernie's Kapha body type.

Dr. Frick's work with the couple was not a hit-or-miss proposition. They tested and counter-tested the biology, followed protocols, and made a strict measurement of the frequencies involved with each potential remedy. Eventually, she worked out Bernie's new meals and treatment plan, a complete diet consisting of whole foods, supplements, and herbs.

Bernie, too, was consulted. As we now know, part of her "magic" is Dr. Frick's ability to communicate with animals. In fact, working in consultation with Bernie sped up the process of figuring out what dietary items would best help him, beginning with established "Yes" and "No" piles that separated (eliminated, really) the non-useful from the useful. The result was a menu plan of correctly measured meals for Bernie that would go inside him and stay in there, leading to less of the tremors and stiffness that had been part of his symptoms when he first arrived at the clinic.

A year later (2019), Bernie was a healthy, vibrant dog in his 11th or 12th year of age. He made a remarkable recovery! The tumor shrunk, too. He outlived every traditional doctor's expectation.

Her experience with Bernie caused Dr. Frick's interest in the Ayurvedic approach to blossom. Uncommonly— unlike others in her line of work, when she studies a subject, she goes at it until she knows the subject COLD.

Dr. Frick addressed her understandings of the three doshas as applied to the dog species while walking with this author along Clearwater Beach in Florida one sunny afternoon in 2019. She casually named off each kind of dog and how the three doshas can be diagnosed and assigned to each dog species. For example,

"Great Pyrenees, St. Bernards
and the like, are easy-going, loving,
nurturing, and they like to lay

*around. They're Kapha. And this
can be seen in their problems of
weight and how they handle solids
and accumulate fluids. They have
slower hearts. But they can be
remedied by eating foods designed
to balance these things and bring a
balance that reduces
inflammations."*

We had just revisited one of the dogs we met on the beach with her owner Ruby when Ava continued with the next dosha description.

*"My son Dalton's one Treeing
Walker Coon Hound, on the other
hand, is a Pitta. He's always on the
move with his attention flicking and
moving everywhere, here and there
... he wants to know stuff all the
time. Pittas are robust, muscled,
fast eaters with faster heart rates,
and possessive, driven, and
intelligent. A Pit Bull is a Pitta
type.*

*"I know this dog, Daisy ...
she's a Pitta; she has a purpose
and a function goin' on all the time.
Interestingly, you don't want to
feed lamb to a Pitta; they do not
like this, because lamb is 'hot'
meat."*

Ava was on a roll. Her pace had picked up, and her eyes lit with interest and excitement as she displayed her description of the third and final dosha, the Vata:

*"Vata's are about air and
motion; they're creative. They like
heat around them – they would like
it here in Florida – and they don't
like cold.*

*"Often, dogs in different
doshas look like their category.
Their bodies reflect these. Like
greyhounds, Dobermans, and
whippets ... all Vatas."*

Doshas also combine, meaning no one is an all-or-none proposition. There are gradients, in which one will be more dominant and the other doshas recessed. One can check the balance of these with each other and note the behavior patterns. Correct diagnoses, however, are more complicated and diverse than at first glance. In other words, there is real science behind Ayurveda, not to mention long years of practice.

Where, then, is this all heading for Dr. Frick and her clinic work?

She will always have a hand in the arena of practical, hands-on care, but there will be changes and expansions. As of December 2018, she made a decision to research the possibility of bringing out a new food line based on Ayurveda. Plans are in the works. If one gets the idea of basic pemmican, similar to those used by the Native American tribes of earlier centuries, one understands the nutritional basis and convenience of such a line of products for animals.

*"These will have to be as perfect as
possible but at an affordable price point.
There are no Ayurvedic-based diets on the
market."*

Then there is her supplement line starting with Frick Formula #1. This is a mineral/vitamin/herb mix designed to match the most common nutritional imbalances of dogs and cats, as seen through the hair-tissue-mineral analysis hair testing she does. This product is currently licensed and on the market, among other formulas in the testing pattern. The plan is to make it available in the near future. According to Frick, *"One-half teaspoon added twice daily to a 40-pound dog's diet should work to balance their bodies."*

Her second book is completed and slated for release in 2020. An instructional guide aimed at teaching other doctors how to interpret hair-tissue mineral analysis, Frick's laboratory testing and its ability to present information to clinicians and animal owners about the nutritional state of their animals will be widely publicized and utilized. Then, too, there is her research on this topic published in September 2017 by the IVC *Journal* of the American Holistic Veterinary Medical Association.

Dr. Frick maintains investment and a position with Electromedical Products International, Inc., home of Alpha-Stim technology. With 19 years invested in this science and its applications to the veterinary market, there are no indications that she plans to back off now.

> *"Of all the tools and gadgets and physiotherapy equipment I have, if I was told I could only have one of them to save the greatest number of lives, hands down, without a blink of an eye, the answer would be Alpha-Stim microcurrent therapy. This device is why we see so many miracles."*

More articles, more books, more teaching, more supplements, new ideas, and business propositions are likely because Dr. Frick doesn't recognize the word "retire."

*"I have seen too many lose purpose in
life when they retire. Suddenly, they go
from having meaning for their days and
people to be with, to having a void. And
then the decline begins. Yes, I could do
with some downtime, a bit more R&R, a
few more dances, and time away. But not
too much. There's a lot that I can and still
want to do, starting first with getting rid of
my Lyme Disease. I want to take back my
bod and it's functions."*

Certainly, Ava's mother Sarah would approve: "Use what you got" is her ingoing saying and practical philosophy. She aligns well with Ava's search for one or more comets on which to hitch her future: "If a frog had wings, he wouldn't bump his butt on the rocks" was her practical philosophic approach to innovative thinking, which she encouraged of each of her daughters.

Almost a motto, Dr. Frick's philosophical statement bears repeating here:

*"There is love, and then there is
unconditional love. This is the 'why' so
many people care for animals. I especially
hear it with dog owners, but it is true. No
matter what the situation, an animal's love
is never about things; it is solely about
YOU.*

"Pure, no-strings-attached love.

*"This is also why people will go to
great lengths to save the animals they love:
the animal ALWAYS loves them back."*

* * *

EPILOGUE: HAPPY TRAILS!

When we are young and curious, it is easy to ask over and over, "Why?" Parents know; they agree this dreaded word repeats *ad infinitum*. Unfortunately, too often, the answer becomes, "Because I said so." Or, "Heck, I don't know!"

Raising Dalton, Ava usually explained just enough detail to answer the question, piece by piece, until her boy either had his answer or quietly abandoned his pursuit of why. She doesn't remember if in her childhood she passed through the age of why or simply bypassed it, only that throughout her lower school and, later, college classes, she accepted the information given to her on face value, believing that it must be so.

"There was not a lot of question
coming from me. I was not looking beyond
the wisdom of the professor."

Fortunately, although well into her veterinary career, she woke up upon her reading nutrition documents, research, and publications written by Dr. Royal Lee (Founder of Standard Process, Inc.). Once again, her mind wondered about life and animals. An adult now, she is still the inquisitive kid, asking, "But, why?"

Her constant curiosity carried across everything she ever learned. She couldn't get enough new materials to read. She no longer cared how many words filled a page, but what those words explained, what they could teach her. No longer would it be enough for her to tell an owner only what was going on or what was happening with their animal. For herself and her clients, she felt the need to figure out the "Whys" and paint a more in-depth picture for their sake and hers.

> *"... [I needed to] ferret out the arsonist, not just put out the fire. Is it a traditionally unseen virus or parasite, or chemicals or heavy metals causing the original insult?"*

Her desire to share what she learned and tested on animals led to another book, (perhaps, others will follow) and to computerized frequency-testing systems that differentiate on a large-scale level organ-system function, and stressors. For her, the expansive study required is all a part of the dance, and she long ago accepted the invitation and subscribed.

> *"All my 'dance' partners are part of this beautiful game of life we all play!*
>
> *"Over my years of dancin', I have found that not everyone hears music the same. Some get the beat and can dance to it, let it flow through their body and mine; others cannot, and some do not even realize there is one! Each country-western song can be a new experience with an unknown partner. The steps, the turns, forward and backward movements, under and around; the sequence of steps he uses, each one is unique, if only to a slight degree.*

"Some dancers are good leaders, some not so; some don't even mind following, now and then. The outstanding dancers would take that as an insult to their skill at being the leader and showing the woman off. Other guys know if they dance with a certain female, they must be prepared to let her lead.

"That's just how it goes in dance, in living, and with animals.

"The year I started ballroom dancing, I was humbled. I thought I was good at the waltz. I love how it sways, and its rhythms and motions, the floating across the dance floor.

"Well, Ballroom ain't Country-Western! The Waltz, Foxtrot, Salsa, Rumba, Cha-cha ... each has a life of its own. For some of them, at my age and having spent years past running and keeping a straight frame, my waggle don't have the wiggle it needs. Nonetheless, learning, experiencing, and allowing my body and mind to be taught differently is still fun.

"If I die without making an effort to teach others, so we can help a higher number of animals to better health, then my time learning what I have will be wasted.

"In that case, shoot, I could have been out ridin,' instead.

*"Now, maybe you've taken hold of a
leash, reins, or a paw and invited an
animal to help you survive, perhaps not.
The answer to that and the result was
always by your choice, your acceptance.
Life and living were, are, and always will
be your adventure, your journey to make
or break.*

*"That choosing, that right to make the
decisions which will determine your
destiny or your fate, remains the core of
not only your heritage as part of
humanity's urge to survive but also the
most profound sense of your being here.
Keep that in mind. Keep your freedoms of
choice intact. Be your own best friend.
And, be kind to animals."*

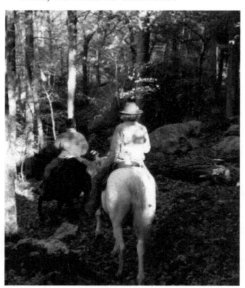

'HAPPY TRAILS UNTIL WE MEET AGAIN!' Dalton & Ava (Mom) riding

* * *

AFTERWORD

Ava Lee Frick—the woman, certified Animal Chiropractor, Doctor of Veterinary Medicine, Mother, Animal Chiropractic Hall of Fame Founding Inductee, "St. Louis' Animal Whisperer," Founder of Pet Rehab & Pain Clinic, philanthropist, published author, lecturer, seminarist, St. Louis Cardinals baseball fan, automobile enthusiast, musician, lover of animals, and a unique spiritual being having a human experience like the rest of us—is a talented and skilled practitioner. Also a communicator extraordinaire, she looks forward to meeting people and sharing with them in person not only her knowledge but more of her anecdotal stories of the animals she has met, communicated with, and fixed up.

For Ava Frick, the future looks endlessly beautiful. We hope that one day you will get to meet her in person, for then you will be forever a part of the rest of her remarkable story!

* * *

ACKNOWLEDGMENTS:
AVA FRICK, D.V.M.

Dalton, my son – you are the light of my life and the reason I am.

Family and Friends – you contributed to my life these past 64 years in so many ways.

Dr. Joseph T. McGinity – my Vet college Large Animal Medicine and Surgery professor, my go-to for moral support in tough times.

My clients – for entrusting me with the life of your individual animals.

All the animals to whom I have ever said, "Thank you."

Ron Kule – this adventure with you was the most successful "marriage" I worked at making go right.

RONALD JOSEPH KULE
Edwin Dearborn – thanks for connecting Ava and me.

Author L Ron Hubbard – always an inspiration to me.

Yulia Varlakhina, my Muse.

SPECIAL ACKNOWLEDGMENT:

To Gus, the "hopeless"10-year-old Cardigan Corgi, who, unable to stand or walk for five years, within 90 days walked and then played joyfully with children for the remainder of his extraordinary sixteen years. What an inspiration you were!

AVA FRICK BOOKS & COURSES:

Fitness In Motion: Keeping Your Equine's Zones at Peak Performance, Lyons Press.

Alpha-Stim® Science, Research, And Animal Applications

Alpha-Stim For Animals – DVD

Chiropractic Stretching Exercises for Horses - (BOOK ON CD)

Clinical Animal Nutrition – DVD

ONLINE: *Advanced Canine Nutrition*

ONLINE: *Fitness In Motion – Stretching and Exercises For Dogs*

Stretching And Exercise For Dogs – DVD

TAI CHI-HUAHUA© - DVD

How to Interpret Hair Tissue Mineral Analysis In Dogs, Cats, and Horses, by Ava Frick, DVM and Maria Wakefield (release in 2020)

HTTPS://WWW.AVAFRICK.COM/

* * *

ABOUT RONALD JOSEPH KULE

Ronald Joseph Kule is an acclaimed author, biographer, novelist, and ghostwriter. Born in Bogota, Colombia, his Polish-American /Colombian-Chilean lineage paint-brushed his life-canvas with a wanderlust and pushed him to visit foreign countries on three continents and deliver keynote engagements and seminars in 17 of them.

Kule appreciates ethnic differences among cultures, having observed directly the disparate societies and conditions of Colombia, Peru, Panama, Chile, China (PRC), Russia, Denmark, Sweden, England, Netherlands, Germany, France, Belgium, Switzerland, Italy, Poland, the Czech Republic, Austria, Luxembourg, Barbados, St. Lucia, St. Vincent, Aruba, Bonaire, Netherland Antilles, the 48 contiguous American states and Hawaii, five Canadian provinces, and Mexico.

The author smiles and laughs easily, often displaying a panoply of emotions; yet, he prefers to make other people happier for having met him or read his books:

"If you curl up with one of my books and find yourself breathless, provoked, inspired, and changed ... and you feel you have undertaken an important journey that left you emotionally satisfied, I will have done my job as your author."

Author Ronald Joseph Kule lives and works in Clearwater, Florida.

* * *

OTHER BOOKS BY

RONALD JOSEPH KULE:

CAROLINA BASEBALL PRESSURE MAKES DIAMONDS, and its eBook, *Pressure Makes Diamonds a Timeless Tale of America's Greatest Pastime* (J. David Miller & Ronald Joseph Kule, 2010) – historical non-fiction.

POETIC JUSTICE ~ *CAROLINA BASEBALL 2012 ~ The Historic Run for the Three-peat* (KuleBooks LLC).

CHEF TELL The Biography Of America's Pioneer TV Showman Chef (Skyhorse Publishing, 2013), Forewords by Regis Philbin & Chef Walter Staib. (Hardcover, Kindle book, and Audiobook.)

LISTEN MORE SELL MORE VOLUME ONE ~ The Anatomy of a Sale; Swedish edition: *LYSSNA MER SAL MER*; Spanish edition: *ESCUCHA MAS VENDE MAS*; Russian edition (late 2020) *БОЛЬШЕ СЛУШАЕШЬ БОЛЬШЕ ПРОДАШЬ КНИГА ПЕРВАЯ: АНАТОМИЯ ПРОДАЖИ.* (KuleBooks LLC) – self-help, non-fiction.

RUINED BY MURDER ADDICTED TO LOVE (KuleBooks LLC, 2014) – mystery/romance novel.

THUNDERCLOUD (The Oddities of a Young Man's Journey to Manhood) (KuleBooks LLC, 2016) – magical realism novel.

HAUNTED ROBOTS (James Patrick Warner & Ronald Joseph Kule, from a story by (the late) Michael E. Noll) (The Haunted Robots LLC, 2018) - a Sci-fi novel.

LIVING BEYOND IMPOSSIBLE ~ The Terry Hitchcock Story, foreword by Tracy Repchuk (KuleBooks LLC, 2019) – biography.

LISTEN MORE SELL MORE VOLUME TWO: The Mechanics of Selling. (KuleBooks LLC, 2019) – self-help, non-fiction.

MINNIE BOLTON'S OLDE VERMONTER RECIPES (with Terry Hitchcock, 2019) – recipes cookbook, non-fiction.

CONVERSATIONS WITH ANIMALS (From Farm Girl to Pioneering Veterinarian ~ Dr. Ava Frick Story), with Dr. Ava Frick, DVM, 2020) – Hybrid Biography, non-fiction.

* * *

For author-signed copies, order through:

HTTPS://RONKULEBOOKS.COM

* * *

SOCIAL MEDIA CONTACT LINKS:

Ava Frick, D.V.M.:

https://www.avafrick.com/

https://www.avafrick.com/shop/

https://www.animalrehabstlouis.com/

email: dravafrick@avafrick.net

Ronald Joseph Kule:

https://www.facebook.com/Ronald.Joseph.Kule/

https://www.facebook.com/KuleBooksLLC/

https://www.facebook.com/BetterEasierSellingTechnol
ogy/

https://www.facebook.com/ron.kule.poet/

email: KuleBooksLLC@gmail.com

MISCELLANEA:
AVA FRICK

Education

FitPAWS® Master Trainer™ Canine Fitness Coach Certificate, 2015

Australian College of Phytotherapy; Certificate in Herbal Phytotherapy, 2005-2006

Advanced Course MET and CES Certificate of Proficiency in Electrotherapy, 2002 & 2003

American Physical Therapy Assoc. (APTA); Building an Aquatics Program, Certificate 2002

American Physical Therapy Assoc. (APTA); Pain Management, Neurology Certificate 2001

Option for Animals Advanced Modules in Animal Chiropractic; Diplomat Level 1998-2002

American Veterinary Chiropractic Association; Certification in Animal Chiropractic,1997

University of Missouri; Doctor of Veterinary Medicine, 1980

Missouri Valley College; Biology, 1973-75

Experience

Pet Rehab & Pain Clinic, Owner

Standard Process, Inc. Veterinary Product Marketing Consultant

Animal Fitness Center, PC, Owner & Founder

Veterinary Medical Director, Electromedical Products International

Animal Rehabilitation Foundation, Inc.

Pet Station, PC, Owner & Founder

Franklin County Humane Society of Missouri

Mountain View Animal Hospital, Phoenix, AZ

Arizona Humane Society, Phoenix, AZ

Suburban Central Animal Hospital, Mission, KS

Publications

Is your broodmare getting the NUTRITION SHE NEEDS?, *Equine Wellness*

Electroceuticals: The Wave of the Future is Now, *American Veterinarian*

JAHVMA, Tissue Mineral Patterns in 564 Dogs. Vol 48

Contentment, The American Institute of Stress

Combat Stress, The American Institute of Stress

Equine Stretching Exercises, Are they Effective? *Journal of Equine Veterinary Science*

Frick & Hethcote. *Fitness in Motion: Keeping Your Equine's Zones at Peak Performance.* The Lyons Press

Microcurrent Electrical Therapy, *Journal of Equine Veterinary Science*

Featured in: *Veterinary FORUM Magazine*, "Re-Thinking Rehabilitation, Is Your Practice Missing Out?"

Featured in: Hands-On Healers, *Horse and Rider*

Research Experience

Applications of Tissue Mineral Analysis in animals, publication in process.

Electromedical Products International, Inc.– Alpha-Stim® clinical applications & research in animals

The University of Missouri, College of Veterinary Medicine Parasitology Dept. 1978 - 1979

Health Industries Department of Ralston Purina Research Farm, nutritional studies 1976

Teaching Experience
Lecture topics: Clinical Animal Nutrition, Chiropractic, Animal Rehabilitation, Microcurrent Therapy, and Electromedicine, Stress and Pain Management, Balancing the Autonomic Nervous System, Caring for the Athlete to the Aging Patient presented to the following groups, associations, and institutions, 2000 – Present:

American Academy of Pain Management

American Holistic Veterinary Medical Association

American Veterinary Chiropractic Association

American Veterinary Medical Association

Central States Veterinary Conference

Chicagoland Veterinary Conference

Illinois Veterinary Medical Association

International Symposium on Rehabilitation and Physical Therapy in Veterinary Medicine

International Veterinary Acupuncture Society

Midwest Veterinary Conference

Missouri Veterinary Medical Association

Western Veterinary Conference

Wild West Veterinary Conference

Media & Online
Instructor for www.e-trainingfordogs.com online courses Certification by CCPDT & IAABC

KXAM, Phoenix, AZ Talk Show Host "Animal Attraction"

www.VoiceAmerica.com On-Line Talk Show Host, 2010- present

Honors/Awards

Animal Chiropractic Hall of Fame, 2015

Fellowship of the American Institute of Stress, 2013

Emeritus Director Award of Franklin County Humane Society, 2008

Hartz® Mountain Corporation Veterinarian of the Year Runner Up, 2006

Franklin County Human Society of Missouri Visionary Award, 2004

International Who's Who of Professionals, 2003

Service Award, C.H.A.M.P. Assistance Dogs, Inc.2002

Certificate of Recognition, C.H.A.M.P. Assistance Dogs, Inc., 2000

Missouri Valley College Honorary Alumni, 1996

Arizona Humane Society Service Award, 1980

Diamond Laboratories Student Service Award, 1980

Who's Who in American Colleges and Universities, 1980

First Woman President, Missouri Student Chapter AVMA, 1979

A. H. Groth Student Research Award,1979

Frank Wells Scholarship, 1979

* * *

A BRIEF HISTORY OF
VETERINARY MEDICINE

Urlugaledinna, the first man ever recorded to have a passion for animals, lived circa 3000 B.C. in Mesopotamia where he expertly healed them. From that time forward, numerous references to "veterinarians" and veterinary practice are found throughout literature.

The founding of a veterinary school in Lyon, France, in 1761 by Claude Bourgelat marks the start of the veterinary profession.

The Odiham Agricultural Society met in 1785 in Hampshire, UK, and resolved, "… the Society will consult the good of the community in general, and of the limits of the Society in particular, by encouraging such means as are likely to promote the study of farriery (horseshoeing, from the Latin *farrerius* and *ferrum* – "iron") upon rational scientific principles." Six years of deliberations followed and established, at last, in 1791, the London Veterinary College, inducing the development of a veterinary science backed by a professional group dedicated to animal medicine.

Initially centered on the horse—a focus that remained for many years influenced by the needs of the Army, over time, the interests of the profession spread to cattle and other livestock, then dogs, and eventually to another category, exotic and pocket animals.

* * * * *

Ava Frick's Cast of Characters

Barn cats, barn cats, and more barn cats

Fanny – the first Pembroke Welsh Corgi

Blossom

A variety of other dogs, none of which were mine

Pilgrim – the bucket calf that got me in to 4H, where I learned to square dance

Pinky – the deaf white cat in Junior High, had a litter of kittens… all died of feline distemper. A difficult lesson.

NeHi, a goat

Punky – male white cat. HBC died the day I returned from visiting Missouri Valley College, Feb 3, 1973

BeGee – from early college for over 19 years, I lived with her more years that all with my parents!

Keoki – Pembroke Welsh Corgi, got as a puppy in Arizona. Over 15 years - delightful and kind dog

Finney – my first English Lop house rabbit that started it all

Amiga – first horse of my own, an Appaloosa

Some finches

Reba, the rat

Skittles, the guinea pig

Joey – a spitz Pekingese mix; showed up one day at about 7 months. Stayed for 17 years… the best ever

Poncey – a quarter horse, taught me to be specific and pay attention to all my body language

Oso – another beautiful English Lop house rabbit

Ralph – the first Vietnamese pot-bellied pig the HSMO had, my first, too

Bart, the goat

Oliver, a cat – loved the baby. Baker, a lovely feline

Chuckie – Dalton's first "pony," a miniature horse

Agnes and Sheeza – other pot-bellied pigs

Twinkie – a Palomino … what a story!

Boogie – a foster corgi we adopted and loved but met a too-early death

Cheerio – a corgi; picked her out the day after Boogie died at Thanksgiving. With us over 15 years.

Mel – my Connemara pony (horse)

Bobaloo – our donkey who loved Fritos and to be photographed

Dalton's fishes

Token - a cat found at a resort during a veterinary conference

Ford, a cat who now lives in Texas with Carmen, another cat, and Frank - a person

Nelson and Clouseau – current cat pets

Dover, whose life is a do-over.

And all of Dalton's hounds and horses

"I apologize to any I may have left out." – **Ava**

* * *

Clinic Note:

Dr. Frick's clinic staff sent this poem with notes to families - another perspective on the passing of a dog friend. Author unknown:

A Dog's Purpose

"God summoned a beast from the fields, and He said, 'Behold man created in my image. Therefore, adore him. You shall protect him in the wilderness, shepherd his flocks, watch over his children, accompany him wherever he may go, even into civilization. You shall be his companion, his ally, his slave.

"To do these things, God said, 'I endow you with these instincts uncommon to other beasts: faithfulness, devotion, and understanding surpassing those of man himself. Lest it impair your courage, you shall not foresee your death. Lest it impair your loyalty, you shall be blind to the faults of man. Lest it impair your understanding, you are denied the power of words. Let no fault of language cleave an accord beyond that of man with any other beast or even man with man. Speak to your master only with your mind and through your honest eyes.

"'Walk by his side; sleep in his doorway; forage for him; ward off his enemies; carry his burden; share his afflictions; love him, and comfort him. And in return for this, man will fulfill your needs and wants, which shall be only food, shelter, and affection.

"'So be silent, and be a friend to man. Guide him through the perils along the way to this land that I have promised him. This shall be your destiny and your immortality.' So spoke the Lord.

"And the dog heard and was content."

* * *

A Sunday Ride in Rural Missouri

This horse ride started in Raymondville,
A quiet Missouri town.
With population 400 some odd
Folk's is always a horsin' around.

Sunday's ride was a follow-up
To Saturdays 25 miler.
Our trail boss had guaranteed
That this one would be shorter.

Now, I want you to know that our trail boss
Was a local cowpoke and trailblazer.
So we had 100% confidence
That he knew where he was about to take us.

There were a total of 15 riders;
10 on gaited, 3 mules, and 2 quarters.
Any horseman knows from odds like that
The last 5 were in for some trottin'.

Three hours past, it's break time at last.
So we stop at a riverbank
For a snack, short rest, and the body's essentials.
Then remount, and we're back on the trail.

We had no idea this was not half-way
Why by lunch that was generally the agenda.
What started out as a short trail ride
Soon became a mission improbable.

Picture yourself at the crest of a hill,
One that's nothin' but rocks.
Below a quagmire, then a dry creek bed.
And beyond? Well, let's say it's a turf never trod.

The hill had to be 60 degrees steep
And a good 1/8 mile long.
Full of thorn bushes, scrub trees, undergrowth and the like
And our only way out was through it!

So through it, we went, like a bunch of ole' goats.
Tho some more willing than others.
Anticipating we were near the end
It was a "do this one for the Gipper."

This alone could have made enough stories
To tell our grandkids about.
But the saga continued, it just wernt' our day.
Listen on, and you'll hear how it ended.

We stopped once to get some directions.
Accurate I was sure they must be,
Except that the leaders missed a crucial turn.
Two hours later, we were back at a familiar tree.

The trek continued through a dry river bed
With foliage and overgrowth thick.
The suns a setting; and I start to prayin',
"Dear Lord, get us outta here quick!"

Our horses don't seem too frazzled.
Tho riders are becoming irate.
It's been six hours since we left camp.
A welcome site would be the farm gate.

Finally, we're at the county highway
And casualties had taken a toll.
One mule was ponied up the mountain.
One horse had thrown a shoe.

With 40-some miles behind us
One local rider said, "What the heck!"

And stopped at the first farmhouse
To call for his truck and rig.

Ten of the 15 riders
Hitched a ride back with him.
Leaving now five of us
To complete the 10 miles to town.

It had been a long day, now the end was in sight.
We were tired and empty our packs.
That day I discovered a drawback to young horses,
Yep, mine trotted all the way back!

* * *

"Some scientists say that by the middle of this century, 15 to 17 percent of 1,103 species under study could be extinct; habitat destruction will bear a big part of the blame." (Veterinary Economics, *Nature* magazine May 2004)

So, what shall we do about that?

* * *

Homage …
by
Ava Frick
(May 21, 2004)

FIREFLIES

Who'll ever notice when the fireflies die?

When there's none left to sparkle on a June summer's night.

When the fields they once hovered

Are all filled with light.

Who'll ever notice when the fireflies die?

*

Who'll ever notice when the fireflies die?

If there are no farms and open spaces,

Nothing left for hiding places.

When even at dark, there is no night.

Who'll ever notice when the fireflies die?

*

Who'll ever notice when the fireflies die?

Without the night's dark backdrop,

To show off their own light,

No one will even notice

That the fireflies have died.

* * * * *

CPSIA information can be obtained
at www.ICGtesting.com
Printed in the USA
LVHW021139301220
675396LV00044B/2151/J